GUIDELINES FOR A VOLUNTARY CANCER ORGANIZATION

ISBN 92-9018-065-X

UICC Technical Report Series – Volume 65

Guidelines for a Voluntary Cancer Organization

Edited by M. A. Wood

International Union Against Cancer
Union Internationale Contre le Cancer

Geneva 1982

UICC PROGRAMME ON CANCER CAMPAIGN & ORGANIZATION
Chairman : Mr. J.H. Young (USA)

WORKSHOP ON GUIDELINES FOR A VOLUNTARY CANCER ORGANIZATION
Geneva, Switzerland, 30 November - 1 December 1981

List of participants

Mr. Michael A. Wood (Chairman)
Director
Ulster Cancer Foundation
40 Eglantine Avenue
Belfast BT9 60X
Northern Ireland

Mr. Raymond Barmont
Secretary General
Ligue Nationale Française
contre le Cancer
1-3 avenue Stephen-Pichon
75013 Paris
France

Mr. Rennie L. Davison
Executive Director
Manchester Regional Committee
for Cancer Education
Kinnaird Road
Manchester M20 9QL
United Kingdom

Dr. Liisa Elovainio
Education Officer
Cancer Society of Finland
Liisankatu 21B
00170 Helsinki 17
Finland

Mrs. Gerry A. de Harven
Director, International Activities
American Cancer Society, Inc
777 Third Avenue
New York, NY 10017
USA

Dr. Olivier Jallut
President, Swiss Cancer League
& President, Association of
European Cancer Leagues - Members
of the UICC
avenue du Théâtre, 7
1005 Lausanne
Switzerland

Mrs. Mirjam Klein
Director General
Israel Cancer Association
P.O.B. 7065
Tel-Aviv
Israel

CONTENTS

PREFACE

In the ten years since the UICC Committee on Cancer Control Programmes published its *Guidelines for a National Organization for Cancer Control* [1], the number of Cancer Leagues and Societies throughout the world has grown significantly and many of the existing organizations have grown considerably in size and scope.

It has become clear that many newly formed Leagues would be happy to have guidance on a suitable structure, ways of raising funds and methodology in the organization of public education campaigns. Other well established organizations may be on the look-out for new techniques or wish to expand into new activities such as the development of a programme of psychosocial support for cancer patients and their families.

Although, these Guidelines have been written primarily for the benefit of the newly established Societies, or those undergoing re-organization, the UICC is sure that the advice they contain will provide new insights and approaches for all but the most sophisticated organizations.

Over the years, the UICC through its Programmes on Education and Cancer Campaign and Organization has produced a number of Guidebooks on various aspects of the work of a Voluntary Cancer League starting with the *Guidelines for a National Organization for Cancer Control* prepared by the Committee on National Cancer Control Programmes. More recently, series of Workshops have been launched to present these documents to the cancer control community in various countries or regions and discuss with Member Organizations ways of adapting these general principles to the constraints of special local circumstances. These Workshops on smoking control, doctor involvement in public education, cancer education in schools, fundraising, etc., have met with a warm reception and have, moreover, provided an insight into the needs of a Cancer Society and a wealth of material to respond to these needs. An attempt has been made to incorporate this experience into these Guidelines.

---

[1] *Guidelines for a National Organization for Cancer Control. Prepared by the Committee on National Cancer Control Programmes of the International Union Against Cancer. 1970. 30 pp. Out of print.*

The UICC has also devoted itself to establishing an Audio-visual Resources Centre for Public Education about Cancer which collects catalogues and disseminates new films, filmstrips, slides, brochures and posters for use in education campaigns. However, on many occasions, advice has been requested as to how programmes should be structured to make the best possible use of the many effective educational aids that are now available. These Guidelines also address themselves to this problem.

Following up our gratifying experience of regional Workshops, it is hoped that over the coming years, various Cancer Societies will be able to organize small meetings of their volunteers and staff to review the various chapters of these Guidelines and, together with various UICC experts, study ways of intensifying or expanding their Society's activities.

INTRODUCTION

Many people throughout the world are working together for a common purpose - a successful attack on cancer. Chances for success are enhanced when maximum "know-how" is combined with the enthusiasm of a group of volunteers, directed toward this common goal.

Most countries have existing cancer control programmes but there are still many which do not yet have a specific cancer society or league. The object of these guidelines is to help existing organizations to examine their structure and activities and to give new organizations an insight into how successfully to implement new programmes.

Although it is difficult to produce a document that will be equally useful for groups at various stages of development in a variety of countries, it is hoped that these guidelines will serve their purpose for all concerned. However it is recognised that not all activities described in the following chapters will be either appropriate or feasible for every voluntary cancer organization.

CHAPTER 1 - ORGANIZATION OF A VOLUNTARY CANCER ORGANIZATION

The same basic organizational structure is common to most cancer societies (leagues or associations), but may of course vary in detail depending on local needs and circumstances.

INTRODUCTION

The majority of cancer societies are initiated by dedicated persons, who realize that a voluntary organization can supplement the basic facilities for the fight against cancer provided by the State. They understand that their individual chances for success in combating cancer will be greatly enhanced if their enthusiasm, expertise and energies are directed through the agencies of a National Cancer Society. Such an organization with comprehensive aims and objectives, will make it possible to achieve maximum impact on the cancer problem in the country.

However, much enthusiasm can be dissipated and valuable time and effort employed ineffectively if, right from the start, the organization's potential aims and objectives are not thoroughly debated and subjected to critical analysis and then drawn up in a clear and concise document that has the unanimous support of all the founders.

1.1.   DEFINITION OF PRIORITIES

The aims of the cancer society can be decided only after careful analysis of available information about the cancer problem in the country. These problems might differ in various regions or local communities. To that end, it will be essential to contact governmental health authorities, medical and paramedical professionals, and other organizations which may have interest in the subject, and who can supply the necessary data.

After all the necessary initial information has been collected, the group must define, as clearly as possible, the aims and objectives of their Society, in various areas of their country. They must also clarify their priorities in respect of their implementation, and decide on the Society's future activities whilst taking a realistic view of the human and financial resources that are likely to be available.

Objectives and programmes should be defined as accurately as possible. This is especially important with a new organization, since policies and programmes will have to be re-examined periodically in the light of local or national experience, and changes made according to the evaluation of their effectiveness.

1.1.1.   Aims and Objectives

The common aims of a cancer society are listed below and in each case specific ways of achieving these aims are suggested:-

1. To initiate, establish, and supplement services and projects in all the fields of the fight against cancer in the country.

<u>Implementation</u>:   - Establishment of treatment and hospitalization centres.

- Acquisition of modern equipment.

- Support of innovative medical programmes.

- Activation of early detection services.

- Establishment of rehabilitation programmes, paramedical and welfare services.

- Support of research.

- Promotion of cancer registry.

2. To involve governments in cancer and cancer-related problems, and to ensure that the subject is dealt with on a national level.

<u>Implementation</u>:   - Liaison with governmental bodies so as to ensure co-operation in anti-cancer activities.

- Promotion of legislation in the fields of carcinogenesis and prevention of cancer.

- Encouragement of governmental allocations for deveopment of anti-cancer services.

- Extension of governmental welfare provision to cancer patients.

3. To ensure the co-operation and involvement of scientists, oncologists, surgeons, physicians, nurses and other health professionals.

<u>Implementation</u>:   - Contacts with medical, health professional, and academic bodies.

- ´Involvement of experts from various areas in the advisory professional committees of the Society.

- Short-term engagement of lecturers and counsellors for public education programmes.

- Action for the inclusion of oncology studies in the curriculum of medical schools.

- Promotion of professional education by conducting symposia, seminars, workshops and congresses, awarding grants for advanced studies, inviting world-renowned experts for visits, etc.

4. To reach the public at large, to broaden its understanding regarding cancer, so as to decrease fear of the disease and prevalent prejudice; and to win the public's co-operation on such vital matters as:
(a) Prevention and early detection of cancer.
(b) Fundraising.

Implementation: - Commission of opinion and attitude surveys.

- Planning of public education and information programmes for specific target groups.

- Smoking control.

- Use of mass-media.

- Production of audiovisual aids, literature, and publications.

- Involvement of the public in anti-cancer voluntary work.

5. To provide a suitable framework for volunteers and professional participants, so as to facilitate the implementation of the Organization's policies and regulations.

Implementation: - Drawing up of a Constitution and Bye-laws, establishing the formal structure of the Society.

- Creation of frameworks for voluntary activity in accordance with the Society's objectives.

- Recruitment of professional and lay volunteers.

- Employment of executive staff.

6. To raise funds for the Organization's activities, as well as for special projects.

Implementation: - Organization of fund-raising programmes.

- Involvement of volunteers in fund-raising projects.

- Publicity.

- Investment of collected funds.

- Budgeting.

- Control and audit of funds raised and expended.

7. To establish close contacts with other national and international cancer organizations thus providing a forum for co-operation on common policies and subjects of mutual interest.

Implementation: - Membership of international cancer organizations.

- Participation in congresses, conventions, and workshops in various parts of the world and hosting of such events.

- Co-operation on international projects of the fight against cancer.

- Current exchange of information and expertise with other organizations.

3

1.2.   CONSTITUTION

Once the aims and objectives of the Organization have been specified, the community to be served has been defined and the legal requirements studied, the Organizing Committee will have to draft the Constitution. The Constitution should define and clarify a number of legal issues:

1.2.1.   *The Society's Institutions*

The Constitution should lay down clearly the formal structure of the Society, and the requirements for meetings of the General Assembly, Council, Executive Committee, and Advisory Panels.

Membership conditions of the Council and Committees must be specified in the Constitution. Members should represent volunteer groups - professionals and laymen - with predetermined proportions to ensure a numerical balance between these groups.

Term of Service. A fixed percentage of the longest serving members should be allowed to retire each year, to make room for new members. These retiring members can be re-elected if the General Assembly so decides.

1.2.2.   *Control of Funds*

Since most National Cancer Societies will be dependent upon contributions and voluntary funds, it is absolutely crucial that the Constitution should establish means for the control of the proper application of these funds. It must also stipulate clearly the different fields of responsibility of the various officials with regard to these funds, and ensure an independent audit in respect of funds raised and expended.

1.2.3.   *Membership*

The Constitution will also have to define types of membership in the Society.

Individual Members: These are persons who join the Society and support it financially or who are given specific tasks.

Corporate Members: Organizations or groups which support the work of the Society. These may also be branches of the National Society in different parts of the country, or Regional Organizations or groups working for a common goal with it.

Persons and organizations who would like to become members of the Society will have to apply to the Council. The Council is free to accept or to reject applicants. The member has to agree to comply with the conditions of membership.

Individual Members and the nominees of Corporate Members are entitled to vote at the General Assembly and are eligible to be elected as Officers or Council Members.

Members will pay a yearly membership fee, determined by the General Assembly on the basis of the recommendations of the Council.

Termination of membership will be implemented according to rules laid down in the Constitution.

National legislation will probably require that Constitution be lodged with a governmental supervisory authority and can be amended only by decision of the General Assembly. It is consequently wise to obtain the assistance of a lawyer in drawing it up, ensure that it is sufficiently wide in scope to cover forseeable expansion of the organisation. Once it has been established, considerable effort and time will be required to modify it.

Some organizations limit their Constitution to the main framework of provisions and then draw up Bye-laws covering detailed administrative points which can be amended by the Council should experience prove it necessary.

A typical draft constitution is given on page 107.

1.3.   *ORGANIZATIONAL STRUCTURE*

The basic pattern of organization suggested here is one which allows physicians, scientists, lay persons, to serve together for a common purpose.

The same basic structure is common in most cancer societies. Though there is variation in detail, depending on local needs, the underlying principle is the same.

At an early stage of the Society's formation, a nucleus of interested people (which should preferably include a number of doctors and scientists) should act as "pace setters". These people must set a personal example and establish all necessary contacts with health authorities and community services, each through his own professional or social organization. The most valuable method of recruitment of additional volunteers is by personal contact, e.g. with a colleague or friend.

It is essential that this group should not seem to favour a single hospital or group of physicians. The non-medical men and women should be recruited from a variety of occupations, economic and educational groups, industry, finance, communication, government, law, philanthropic societies, etc.

Out of this group the Organizing Committee will be established. At this time, informal meetings for policy-making will be held. This will lead at a later stage to the development of a well-defined structure for the running of a constantly growing cancer control organization.

In larger countries, or as the size and strength of the organization increase, it may be necessary to establish a regional structure by which the national society stimulates the establishment of local groups in large cities or other population centres. However, it is essential that the national society continue to exercise close overall supervision, provide training and exercise programme support functional in accordance with policy laid down by the Council and the relevant committees.

The organizational structure should be pyramidical and built on the following lines:

- General Assembly
- Council
- Committees
- Officers
- Staff
- Control of Funds

All these subjects will be dealt with in detail in the following pages.

1.3.1.   *General Assembly*

The General Assembly is made up of all individual members and authorized representatives of corporate members.

This body is, in fact, the "shareholders' meeting", and the powers of the Society are vested in it.

The General Assembly will convene once in each calendar year. Members will be invited according to rules provided in the Constitution.

The suggested tasks of the General Assembly are as follows:-

- To receive reports on activities of the Council.
- To discuss and approve financial and activity reports presented.
- To appoint auditors.
- To elect the officers of the Society. These are usually:

    Patron

    President

    Vice-Presidents

    Chairman of the Council and Executive Committee

    Vice-Chairmen

    Secretary General

    Treasurer

- To elect the Council and the Executive Committee.

In some societies the power to elect the officers, Executive and Advisory Committees are delegated to the Council.

In that case, the General Assembly will elect the Members of Council only.

1.3.2.   *Council*

Although the Council is normally elected by the General Assembly, it may precede the Assembly in the process of formation of a new Cancer Society.

The Council is initially formed from suitable volunteers, representatives of the different groups involved in the establishment of the Society. It is the major governing body of the Society. It will, as a primary task, draw up a draft Constitution, for approval by the General Assembly.

Council membership will be elective with new members, proposed at the Annual Meeting of the General Assembly.

Since the Council is likely to consist of a large number of people, they will confine themselves usually to consideration of general programmes and projects proposed, and to determination of general policy, leaving details to Committees. The Council will usually appoint the Chief Executive of the Cancer Society. (See also *Executive Committees 1.3.3.*)

Because the Council may be too large a body for the day-to-day administration of the Society, it will often delegate some of its powers to one or more executive committees.

The number of Executive and Advisory Committees appointed will depend on the range of the Society's activities and in smaller societies the responsibilities of one or more committees may be combined.

Committees initiate programmes of their own, but may also receive and check requests for assistance and funds from various agencies, physicians, scientists, educators etc with new ideas for projects that could advance cancer control programmes.

Members of the Committees should include volunteers – professional and laymen – and in certain circumstances, staff. Interaction among the various Committees should be encouraged. One good way of achieving this is by involving Advisory Committee Chairmen in the Executive Committees and Councils as well.

Minutes to be signed by the Chairman should be kept at all Committee meetings.

The Chairman of the Council may serve simultaneously as the Chairman of one of the Executive Committees.

1.3.3.   *Executive Committees*

Executive Committees are different from all other committees in that they have fixed responsibilities delegated by the Council, while other committees have only advisory functions.

Executive Committees should implement policy within the scope of their responsibilities either in consultation with or after recommendations from the various advisory committees.

An important function of one of the executive committees, which will usually be designated as the Finance Committee, will be the control of finances including the preparation of budgets, ensuring that money is spent prudently and that proper accounting procedures are carried out and full financial reports made to Council.

Other important functions of executive committees will be the planning and initiation of fundraising campaigns, the appointment of staff and monitoring of their activities (see also *1.3.2.*) and the general control of the society's programmes.

Since committee activities will range over many fields it may be necessary to appoint sub-committees. In any case, executive committees should meet at regular intervals to ensure the smooth running of the Cancer Society.

1.3.4.   Advisory committees

The number of specific responsibilities of advisory committees will depend again in a large measure upon the variety of the activities in which the Cancer Society is involved. They will be appointed to advise Council and the executive committees on specific aspects of the society's programmes and the needs which exist in the community. The following committees are likely to be required by most cancer societies involved in a comprehensive approach to the cancer problem.

1.3.4.1.   Committee on Health Care

This Committee's responsibility will be to advise on all programmes for early detection and medical services in the field of cancer, including the allocation of funds for early detection services; the development and expansion of cancer treatment centres, with particular emphasis on construction and the acquisition of equipment; and the implementation of innovative medical programmes. These activities must of course be co-ordinated with the official health authorities, either national or local. Members will include: physicians (especially oncologists), medical-service planning experts, government representatives, financial advisors.

1.3.4.2.   Committee on Research

Its responsibility will be to advise on the support of cancer research at universities, research institutes and hospitals. Its membership should include representatives from all the disciplines in which research applications might be made although applications for research funding may be referred to outside referees.

1.3.4.3.   Committee on Service, Welfare and Rehabilitation

Its responsibility will be to advise the Society on the planning and supervision of programmes aimed at assisting cancer patients and their families. Membership will include: social workers, physicians, nurses, community and religious leaders and representatives of voluntary organizations.

1.3.4.4. (i)   Committee on Public Education and Information

This Committee will advise on the development of the public
education programmes, (a) to change peoples' fear of cancer to a
more realistic and hopeful view. (b) to bring cancer patients to
physicians in earlier stages of the disease. (c) to publicise
the Society's programmes.

In larger cancer organizations it may be advisable to divide
responsibility between two committees, one dealing with public
education and information; and the other with public relations.

In this case there has to be close interaction between the
two Committees. For suggested membership see Chapter 5, Education
and Information Programmes.

1.3.4.4. (ii)   Committee on Professional Education

The task of this Committee will be to determine ways of
supplying to physicians, dentists, nurses and other health
professionals regular information about cancer diagnosis and
treatment, and to advise on how to develop the professional education
programmes of the organization. For suggested membership see
Chapter 5, Education and Information Programmes.

1.3.4.5.   Committee on Smoking Control Activities

In view of the special importance of this subject and the
wide and growing awareness of the health hazards involved in
smoking it may be advisable to establish a separate Committee on
the subject.

This Committee will have to work in close co-operation with
all the other advisory committees concerned and must co-ordinate
its activities accordingly.

Membership should include: physicians, scientists, health
educators, teachers, journalists, business and trade union leaders,
clergy and leaders of voluntary organizations and any other
interested members of the community.

1.3.4.6.   Inter-Committee Communication

All Committees will channel their advice to the relevant
Executive Committees and the Council.

If the Society is to function smoothly and effectively, it
is essential that there be co-ordination among the various advisory
committees in order to prevent a policy being advocated by one
committee and opposed by another. The likelihood of this happening
can be minimized by having members serve on more than one committee
on related subjects.

The participation of chairmen of the advisory committees as
members of one or other of the executive committees is a useful
way of ensuring co-ordination and implementation of policy, and
will enable them to be part of the final decision-making machinery.

The General Assembly or the Council as the case may be, will be required to elect the following officers of the Society. These officers will normally be elected for one year or any defined number of years as decided by the Assembly. They may be re-elected for an agreed number of terms.

<u>Patron</u>: Some cancer societies may wish to appoint a Patron, who could in fact be the Ruler, Sovereign, or President of the State. The Patron may give his or her patronage to important activities on the national level, such as a public education or fundraising campaign.

<u>President</u>: The interpretation of this title varies considerably between the different organizations. It is often an honorary title bestowed upon a distinguished and well-known personality in the community or of the medical profession who has agreed to dedicate his or her support to the Society.

The main function of this office is to represent the Society in high-level gatherings and also to open doors to senior government officers which might otherwise remain closed to the Society's representatives. The President may take part ex-officio in meetings of all committees according to his or her wishes, and will usually chair the Annual General Meeting of the Society.

<u>Vice-Presidents</u>: are similarly appointed and there is usually no set limit to the number of Vice-Presidents in an honorary capacity. It is desirable to elect one of the Vice-Presidents to serve as first Vice-President, who shall act for the President in his or her absence.

Each of these officers shall be eligible for re-election.

<u>Chairman</u>: Acts as Chairman of the Council, and provides policy and programme leadership.

In some cancer societies, the Constitution provides that the Chairman shall be a non-medical member of the Council, but of course he may be a medical professional or scientist if the Council so decides.

<u>Vice-Chairman</u>: It is important that the Vice-Chairman has a different professional background from the chairman. This will ensure the objective and smooth running of the Society.

<u>Secretary-General</u>: Calls meetings, prepares the agenda, maintains the official records of the Society and is responsible for the minutes of the Council. (May in some societies be the Chief Executive).

<u>Treasurer</u>: Supervises the preparation of the annual budget, makes financial reports and supervises the handling of funds, and other assets of the Society.

The office of Secretary and Treasurer may be combined in one person.

The success and effectiveness of the Cancer Society will depend to a large extent on the personality of the Chief Executive, and indeed on the staff as a whole.

Chief Executive: He or she must be a good administrator with a good working knowledge of the fields of service, in which the Cancer Society is involved, be flexible and yet persistent; capable of communicating with people on different levels and with the mass media.

Much of the accomplishment of the volunteers serving the Society will depend on the calibre of the top Staff Executive.

For the success of the Organization it is of utmost importance to avoid conflicts in authority between the Chief Staff Executive and the Society's officers, Council and Executive Committees. This question will normally be resolved in practice, by the exercise of tact and understanding. Obviously determination of policy and programmes belongs to the Council and Executive Committees, but the opinion and advice of the Chief Staff Executive must be taken into account in arriving at those decisions.

No one person could, of course, be an expert in every one of the Society's programmes, specialist professional staff will therefore be needed in addition to the Chief Executive.

Supportive and professional staff may include the following:

- Physicians
- Nurses
- Social Workers
- Psychologists
- Public Relations Officers
- Teachers
- Health Educators
- Accountants
- Secretaries etc.

The number of staff members and their qualifications will depend on programmes operated and funds available. It should always be remembered however that the number of administrative staff should be kept to a minimum in order that expenses will not be excessive. Staff members should be selected not only for their experience, but also for their enthusiasm in relation to cancer control and in their ability to work effectively with volunteers. It is highly desirable that all staff should be non-smokers.

1.4.   CONTROL AND USE OF FUNDS

The proper control and allocation of funds is absolutely crucial. In the outlines of the Constitution there should be definite rules on proper usage of the funds of the Society.

The funds will be expended according to the annual budget presented by the Finance Committee. This budget should have been prepared on the basis of priorities and recommended by the various advisory committees. It will also include the necessary provision of funds for the permanent and current responsibilities undertaken by the Society within its declared policy of aims and objectives.

The budget should be balanced and fundraising campaigns should be planned accordingly. (See Chapter 8, Fundraising).

Reserve funds, if they exist, may help the Executive Committee in accepting responsibility for the planning of larger projects. They also enable the Society to match the financial obligations undertaken by contributors for major, earmarked projects.

The responsibility for the management and control of funds may be executed along the following lines:

(1)   Treasurer: Supervises the preparation of the annual budget and financial reports and supervises the handling of funds.

(2)   Finance Committee: Its task is to approve and/or prepare budgets, to ensure the prudent disbursement of funds and to control investments.

(3)   Accountant or an Accounting Division within the framework of paid staff: Maintains the records and provides information required by the Treasurer and Finance Committee.

(4)   Audit: The Balance Sheet and Financial Report should be approved and signed by an independant certified accountant.

All the above measures are advisable for the smooth running of the Society's financial affairs and as evidence of proper management of public money.

CHAPTER 2 - THE VOLUNTARY CANCER ORGANIZATIONS
CONTRIBUTION TO HEALTH CARE

Different countries of the world have different health care systems, including national health insurance plans, private health insurance plans and special health programmes for lower income groups. Whatever the system, there will never be adequate funds to provide ideal treatment and care facilities for all cancer patients. Especially in countries where cancer is not considered a high priority in the overall national health care programme, the local or national cancer league can provide assistance in many ways.

Existing detection, treatment and aftercare facilities should be reviewed to determine where the greatest needs exist, and recommendations should be made on how these facilities can be improved. Obviously, collaboration with other medical and health organizations, and with appropriate government authorities, is essential. Wasteful duplication must be avoided. Although other local health concerns may seem of greater magnitude, the voluntary cancer league has a duty to its supporters to concentrate on its own special goals and obligations - those of developing adequate prevention, detection, treatment and other services for the control of the disease.

There are three main components of cancer care: organization, personnel and facilities. Each is important, but the first two are more important than the third. The greatest emphasis must be placed on organization, and the training of personnel. Without an efficient organization of trained physicians and supporting personnel, the best facilities are of little value. Even in a community with limited facilities, well trained medical and other health professionals can provide a high standard of cancer care; the best facilities will be useless without them. Of course, when the trained personnel also have the best facilities and equipment to work with, the result will be the best possible treatment for the cancer patient.

The cancer society may therefore decide to provide financial support for such projects as fellowships for training medical and non-medical personnel, construction of facilities for treatment or aftercare programmes, purchasing of equipment, etc. However, all related costs must be analysed and clearly understood. These will include running costs, the salaries of personnel, etc., and a time limit should be set for transferring the financial responsibility from the cancer society to the institution concerned. Such arrangements should be specified in writing and agreed by all concerned. This is necessary to safeguard the society from assuming a major ongoing financial burden that would indefinitely limit its scope and activities in other fields.

2.1.   *GRANTS FOR THE PROVISION OF EQUIPMENT*

Cancer societies can expect to receive applications for grants to purchase apparatus for clinical or research purposes. In each case it is important for the appropriate Committee to investigate

the circumstances surrounding the application. Firstly a
preliminary survey should be carried out to establish that similar
equipment does not already exist in the region, and also that the
same application has not been submitted to another organization.
The Committee must also satisfy itself that the apparatus
concerned is the most suitable for the purpose, what its working
life will be and that it will not be obsolete within a short period
of time. If the results of its enquiries are favourable the
Society should then consult the relevant Hospital/Research Institute
authorities to confirm that any running costs involved in the
acceptance of the apparatus will be met by that authority before
finally approving a grant to the applicant.

Review Committees should fully understand the need for
careful scrutiny and the establishment of priorities in considering
grant applications. Independent experts should be consulted where
necessary. It has happened in some centres that large grants for
sophisticated scientific equipment with all the implied prestige
have been approved, whilst other quite modest applications for
much needed, but more mundane equipment have been turned down.
(See also Chapter 3 - The Scope of Cancer Research).

Because it is unlikely that there will ever be adequate funds
to meet every application, the Society should apply the same
priorities to grants that have already been decided for the
Society's own programmes. It should also be understood that
equipment which directly benefits cancer patients should have
priority over other apparatus.

To Summarize:

The cancer society's role in developing health care programmes
for the cancer patient include:
- a detailed survey of existing programmes for detection,
  treatment and aftercare;
- an analysis of how improvements in the programme can be
  provided within the existing national health care system;
- an evaluation of priorities: what needs are most important;
- an evaluation of the cost-effectiveness of a financial
  commitment from the cancer society, the type of commitment
  and its duration; and
- of most importance: close collaboration with other medical,
  health and especially governmental authorities.

CHAPTER 3 - THE SCOPE OF CANCER RESEARCH

One important activity of many cancer leagues and societies is to provide funds for research. Decisions about the usefulness or otherwise of applications for funding from research workers should of course be made on the recommendations of a panel of doctors and scientists who are familiar with the field of work in which each grant application is made. (See also *2.1. GRANTS FOR THE PROVISION OF EQUIPMENT*).

Even though Committee members who are not medically or scientifically trained may rightly feel unqualified to judge the merits of some research proposals, they should have a general idea of the different areas and scope of research work so that they can talk intelligently about the Society's activities to members of the public who ask them. The range of problems to be solved is vast, absorbing the attention of a host of research workers trained in many branches of medicine, pure science, and the social sciences. Though it would be impossible to describe here in detail what researchers are doing, the following broad outline of the more important fields of research, and the perspectives and manner of approach of specialists working in these fields, may help towards a better understanding of what is implied in the familiar term "cancer research". ·

3.1.   *CANCER IN THE POPULATION*

Epidemiology is the branch of medicine which examines patterns of health and disease in whole populations. Comparison of the number of cases of cancer of different types which occur in different countries, or in different regions of the same country, has shown such striking differences that it can only be concluded that cancer is strongly linked with the environment.

By gathering information about the patterns in which cancer occurs, epidemiologists have not only provided a greater understanding of the nature of cancer but have also been able to identify groups of people - for instance workers in some industries - who are more likely than others to develop some forms of cancer. In turn, this has shown how such cancer can be prevented by removing harmful substances or by protecting workers from them. Very similar methods produced the massive weight of evidence that cigarette smoking causes lung cancer in some people, and pointed the way in which a huge reduction in the present mortality from cancer can be achieved by changing the way people behave.

Epidemiologists also help in research work to find out how best to provide regular health checks for people who may develop

---

This chapter is based on an original publication "Cancer Research" of the former British Cancer Council.

cancer. The cervical smear test (or Pap test) is one example of this kind of screening programme.

Cancer Registries also use the epidemiologists' skills to help assess the results of treatment, and the general quality of life afterwards, of large numbers of cancer patients.

3.2. FINDING THE CAUSES OF CANCER

3.2.1. Carcinogenesis

The process by which cancers are produced is called carcinogenesis. Bearing in mind that the cancers are a group of related diseases, it is only to be expected that they are triggered off in various ways. Many things that can cause cancer in man are already known; and this knowledge, by enabling those who may be at risk to be protected, has resulted in the prevention of certain forms of the disease.

Radiation of various kinds - often used to cure cancer - can actually cause the disease when its use is not controlled. Those doctors who first treated patients by X-rays early in this century often got skin cancer themselves. They did not realise that, being inadequately protected, they were constantly receiving small amounts of radiation which added up to a dose that was dangerous. More recently, many of those who survived the atomic bomb explosions developed leukaemia - sometimes years later. The ultra-violet radiation in sunlight can cause skin cancer. This is a particular risk for fair-skinned people who work out of doors constantly in very strong sunlight in the tropics. And everyone should avoid excessive sun-bathing for the same reason.

Some chemicals can cause cancer. As early as the 18th century, Dr Percival Pott in England noticed that chimney sweeps, who as boys had to climb inside chimneys and sweep them out by hand, developed cancer of the skin through excessive exposure to soot. Two centuries later, the actual chemicals present in coal tar, which can cause cancer in laboratory animals were identified. Other chemicals used in industrial processes are potentially dangerous, but workers can now be protected from them in various ways. Some of the chemicals that have been proved in the laboratory to cause cancer are certainly present in tobacco smoke. In fact, a great number of chemical compounds have now been shown to produce cancer in laboratory animals.

But it is still not known how much human cancer is caused by chemicals in the environment.

3.2.2. Virology

Viruses are also important, because certain viruses cause cancer in animals. The association between viruses and cancer is a special study in itself.

Over the past sixty years, more and more kinds of cancer in a wider range of animal species, ranging from chickens to monkeys, have been shown to be caused by viruses. This has not yet been shown to be true of human cancers; but evidence is beginning to accumulate that some cancers in some people may be due to viruses. The great difficulty of this work is that a suspected virus cannot be administered to *people* to see if they develop cancer. Such evidence about viruses and human cancer is therefore circumstantial and indirect.

It must be said, however, that any viruses involved in the human disease must be quite different in their effect on a community from those viruses that are spread from person to person in epidemics like influenza. If this were not so, doctors and nurses who care for people with cancer would themselves get cancer more frequently than the general population. In fact, they do not.

One of the aims of this kind of research is to gather enough evidence linking viruses to the cause of some forms of human cancer, to justify an all-out effort to develop a vaccine - like polio or influenza vaccine - which would then help to control and prevent any human cancers that are caused by viruses.

3.3.   IMPROVING OUR DEFENCES

3.3.1.   Immunology

Another important line of research is based on the fact that everyone has built-in defences against many diseases, including cancer.

Immunology is the study of the body's natural resistance to foreign organisms. This includes the body's response to its own cells which have become cancerous.

Cancer cells differ from normal cells in many ways. One way in which they differ is that many cancer cells carry distinctive markers, called antigens, on their surface. Cells carrying these markers are recognised by the body as enemies, much as an escaped prisoner who failed to find a change of clothing would be recognised. Normally the body reacts against cells carrying these antigens, and produces what is called an immune response which suppresses, or even destroys, the cancer cells. In very much the same way the body reacts to infectious diseases like measles or diphtheria, and in these cases immunization can increase the body's immune response from these diseases, and so prevent them.

Ways have yet to be found of immunising the body against its' own cancer, but methods of boosting the defence system of some patients are being developed. This research, still in its very early stages, has already been useful in dealing with remaining pockets of cancer cells which conventional methods of treatment have failed to reach.

Another promising and very important line of research is concerned with the study of the blood of patients with cancer to see if any measurable immune reactions are taking place early in the disease. If, as seems likely there are, it would offer the possibility of detecting the presence of cancer long before it begins to cause symptoms, and thus make the early diagnosis of cancer, on which successful treatment so often depends, so much easier.

17

Surgery cures thousands of people of cancer. Another well-established and for some forms of cancer, highly successful method of treatment is by radiation - called radiotherapy. A newer method is chemotherapy - the treatment of cancer by drugs and medicine. All of these treatments are constantly being refined and improved through the efforts of research workers and clinicians from every branch of science and medicine.

3.4.1. *Radiation biology*

Radiation biology is the study of the effects of radiation on living organisms. This includes the effects of radiation on cells - both normal and cancerous. When cancer patients are treated with radiation, and about half of all patients are, cancer cells are destroyed by carefully directed beams of penetrating rays in dosages that are precisely calculated according to the position and size of the cancer. The aim of radiation biologists is to make this treatment even more effective. Bigger doses of radiation destroy more cancer cells, but they also do more damage to the patient's healthy tissue. So the task is to find ways of making either the cancer cells more sensitive to radiation, or the normal cells less sensitive.

The sensitivity of both cancer and normal cells is influenced by the intensity of the radiation and by the length of time over which the treatment is given. A series of relatively small doses is often more effective than one single big one. Radiation treatment is also often more effective when given together with certain drugs and chemicals, called radiation sensitizers. More information is needed about these modifying agents, especially about the possible benefits of combining them with radiation treatment so that the greatest damage to the cancer cells can be achieved without doing too much harm to the normal tissue. Modern research in radiation biology is mainly aimed at solving these problems.

3.4.2. *Cancer chemotherapy*

Cancer chemotherapy is the use of chemicals that are especially destructive to cancer cells. These chemicals, which may be given as tablets or by injection, dissolve in the blood and are carried throughout the body, killing any cancer cell with which they come into contact. Chemotherapy is important because it is the only means so far available for treating cancer that has spread throughout the body. This is the case with the leukaemias, and with solid cancers that have not been entirely removed by surgery or destroyed by radiation at an early stage of their growth.

In recent years important progress has been made and some cancers are now completely cured by chemotherapy. For other cancers the search is still on. Chemicals are tested for their anti-cancer properties in the laboratory, and the chemical make-up of tumour cells is explored to see if they differ in any way from normal cells. In this way it is hoped to develop particular chemicals which might destroy cancer cells without doing permanent damage to normal, healthy cells. This is a problem that complicates cancer chemotherapy as it does radiotherapy. As in most kinds of cancer research, advances in chemotherapy usually come not from dramatic discoveries but from a steady increase in knowledge of cancer, together with painstaking assessment of different methods of treatment, sometimes using combinations of drugs, and sometimes X-rays and surgery together with chemo-therapy.

3.4.3.   *Clinical trials*

Much of the experimental work in developing new methods of treatment is done first of all on laboratory animals. However, the time must finally come when, after repeated laboratory trials, and careful consultation between scientists and doctors, a highly promising line of new treatment must be used on human patients. This is a very important area of research, and it is governed by strict codes of conduct that are now followed by doctors and scientists all over the world.

Clinical trials are carried out to make sure what is the best possible way of treating people suffering from particular forms of cancer. In the past, clinical trials were often undertaken by individual doctors dealing with relatively small numbers of patients. This had·several disadvantages, including the fact that the numbers were too small to allow valid conclusions to be drawn. As a result, there was often very considerable delay in the introduction and general acceptance of even the most worthwhile treatment. Nowadays doctors and research workers recognise that the problems can be tackled more efficiently by close collaboration between interested clinicians and the major cancer treatment centres in controlled clinical trials. By including large numbers of patients in these trials, sometimes from many different centres and countries, and by using modern statistical methods, the statistician can very rapidly offer an accurate assessment of the value of any new treatment, method or technique.

But in all this, the rights and dignity of individual patients must be safeguarded. Nothing that smacks of 'experiment-ation' can be permitted, and in many countries special ethical committees scrutinise every proposal to hold a clinical trial with great care before they allow it to go ahead.

The result is that there is now widespread acceptance of controlled clinical trials at national and international level. These have furthered knowledge of the disease, not only by showing beyond doubt the best kind of treatment for some cancers, but also by improving communications between laboratory research workers and clinicians. As a result, it can be said that modern clinical trials have, to a very great extent, revolutionised the approach to the treatment of cancer.

3.5.   CANCER RESEARCH AND THE PUBLIC

Cancer research does not end with the wide range of activities in laboratories and hospitals. A great deal of vital research goes on, and much remains to be done, into the social aspects of cancer. Epidemiology has already been described. Social research and educational research also have substantial contributions to make in the total attack on the cancer problem.

3.5.1. *Social research*

Applying the social sciences to problems linked with cancer is not new, but it has only recently begun to gather momentum. Why do people behave in ways they would not ordinarily do when faced with signs that are linked in their minds, rightly or wrongly, with cancer? Why do they carry on with harmful habits - such as cigarette smoking - long after everyone knows about the dangers? How is it that bizarre unscientific beliefs about causation persist in the face of modern education? Why does unreasoning fear of cancer remain so little unchanged after years of improving cure-rates?

The attitudes of doctors, nurses and other professionals affect the people, both sick and well, with whom they come in contact. The influence may not always be beneficial, though its potential for good is immense. How can training and day-to-day professional habits be altered to achieve this? These are a few of the subjects that social research examines. All have the practical aim of enabling people to make the best possible use of the preventive and curative facilities already available.

3.5.2. *Educational research*

"When will we find a cure for cancer?" is a question many people ask. The answer is that research *has* found cures for many common forms of cancer, and many thousands of people are completely cured every year. But many thousands more could be if only they saw their doctors soon enough. And even more cancers could be prevented if among other things, people were to stop smoking, chewing betel quid, and if more women were to take advantage of the Pap smear test.

Epidemiological research helps to identify classes of people who are most likely to get cancer - like smokers. Social research reveals why some people do not see the doctor soon enough, or do not take advantage of preventive measures.

Educational research takes these findings and then tries to discover how best to create a greater understanding of the cancers as a group of diseases of which many are now curable, some preventable, and others manageable even though cures for these are not frequent. This involves, among other things, finding ways of getting rid of needless fears and substituting more hopeful, less emotional attitudes to cancer. Public education about cancer has already had some successes: with more research in this area it is hoped to reduce deaths from cancer by many thousands a year. (See also Chapter 5 - Education and Information Programmes).

CHAPTER 4 - SERVICE, WELFARE AND
REHABILITATION PROGRAMMES

INTRODUCTION

Until quite recently services to patients was limited to general services such as transportation and the provision of hospital amenities which were also available to non-cancer patients. In the last twenty years or so however, the treatment of cancers has improved so that many more patients have their cancers either cured or controlled for long periods of time. Such success however was often as a result of fairly severe treatment sometimes involving extensive surgery. Medical teams became more aware of the fact that treatment could not be considered as completed when the patient had been successfully operated on for his cancer. New and difficult problems were arising for the patient who sometimes had to adapt himself to a specific physical handicap which necessitated drastic changes in his personal habits; for instance eating, speaking, breathing and walking. The general management of the result of such therapy has made tremendous progress and such patients can now be helped more efficiently in their rehabilitation to normal life. The progress which has been achieved in rehabilitation of cancer patients has been made possible not only by the work of the health-care team but also by the collaboration of the patients themselves, and self or mutual support groups. This major step forward in helping cancer patients has shown them that it is possible to recover to be active and to live much as they did before treatment. There are several different types of volunteers working in service, welfare and rehabilitation programmes. These include:

1. Devoted people who give part of their time to the community, to the hospital and to patients in general.

2. Patients and patients' families acting as volunteers to help cancer patients, either by making domiciliary calls or at the hospital.

3. Treated cancer patients who will give part of their specific experience to other fellow patients who have had the same treatment and the same problems of adaptation and rehabilitation to normal life.

4.1. *PATIENT SERVICE AND WELFARE PROGRAMME*

There are many ways of helping cancer patients and their families, both in the hospital or at home. The methods described in this chapter are not exhaustive and should only be taken as an example of what can be done. It is important to know local conditions before organizing a volunteer programme.

In order to avoid any conflict of competence with hospital services, medical staff, nurses, or social services, every action which the cancer society initiates to help patients should be well co-ordinated and acceptable to all the health care professionals involved.

Voluntary cancer organizations will receive requests for information and help so it is most important that they are equipped to cope with enquiries from both the patient and relatives. These enquiries may be of matters of a purely practical nature, but it is important to realise that social and emotional needs, though not always discussed, may be as important to the enquirer as the practical problem about which the enquiry is made. As the cancer society may well have to answer very specific questions it is necessary to have competent staff and well-informed, trained volunteers, skilled in both face-to-face and telephone counselling.

4.1.1. *Financial Aid*

This important aspect of services is often one of the justifications given to fund-raising campaigns. It is impossible to give strict guidelines because local conditions and official aid available will vary so much from country to country but even with optimal insurance or health service facilities numerous personal problems of a financial nature will arise. These may vary from sick room supplies and equipment for home use to the support of impoverished families. Any financial help given has to be well organized and the cancer society should have a special committee which will review applications and approve grants. The team will need to be composed of physicians, nurses and social workers as well as administrators from the cancer society in order to be able to judge the validity of the request. It is important that the cancer society has some restrictive criteria on such applications otherwise this one area of support alone could swallow up all the funds that their volunteers are capable of raising.

4.1.2. *Volunteer Help in the Hospital*

Volunteers can organize a service to visit lonely patients in hospital and give them their friendship and the comfort of having another human being to talk to. One solution that has been worked out in the United States of America is through the CanSurmont organization which is described later in this chapter. It is also valuable for volunteers to organize the provision of comforts for patients in hospital and here they should work closely with hospital staff to ensure that appropriate needs are met. There is also need for a recreational team to help keep patients active during their convalescence. Volunteers may also run a hospital shop or library.

4.1.3. *Volunteer Help Outside the Hospital*

There is a clear need in many countries for private transport to be available to bring patients to and from the doctor, hospital or clinic. This is a service which is very adequately operated by volunteers; not only is a driver required but a companion to help with the patients. Whenever possible, volunteers should use their own vehicles rather than that the society should provide funds for the hire of transport. Careful planning of the whole transportation service is essential (i.e. liaison with local health authorities, volunteer training, liability insurance, etc).

4.1.4. *Volunteer Help in the Home*

Volunteers can also help disabled patients in the home; house keeping, minding children, cooking, feeding patients, helping them to dress and giving them support while they are learning to walk etc. Such a service would also need to include the loan or donation of equipment such as special beds, walking aids, crutches, prostheses, etc. It follows that there needs to be a proper storage, distribution, recovery and repair service for such equipment.

4.2. *REHABILITATION PROGRAMMES*

Rehabilitation assists the patient to return to his community occupation and family, able to function as far as possible as before. Any such service must also include help to direct the patient to the means of obtaining such a service. It should also include occupational therapy.

4.2.1. *Mutual Support Groups*

For patient and family the diagnosis of cancer still provokes fear, uncertainty, confusion and loneliness, and the ability to share the sorrow and doubts of other cancer patients will be of great help. There are many mutual support groups working in various ways in different countries. Many are supported by the local cancer society. In Finland, for instance, a general association of all cancer patients operates under the aegis of the Cancer Society of Finland. In the United States there are two important examples of mutual support groups, the "I CAN COPE" programme and the "CanSurmont" programme. However, some groups are spontaneous associations of cancer patients who are dissatisfied with the care which they are receiving, and react against conventional treatment. They may be open to manipulation by unorthodox practitioners and the cancer society has an obligation to help them.

4.2.1.1. *"I CAN COPE" Programme*

The primary purpose of the I CAN COPE programme is to offer information and education about cancer and its treatments and about the effects of the disease, both physically and emotionally, on the patient and his family, and to suggest ways of overcoming the problems and difficulties that ensue. A secondary benefit of the programme is that it offers a built-in support system. Not only do the participants gain a better understanding of their disease, but they also have an opportunity to meet with medical personnel and with other people who are experiencing similar problems and concerns. The I CAN COPE programme is for persons and their families who are experiencing and who are experienced in cancer. The eight sessions or training classes that are offered on a community basis or at a local hospital include the following:

1. Course Introduction.

2. Learning About Your Disease.

3. Learning to cope with your daily health problems.

4. Learning to express your feelings about your disease.

5. Learning to like yourself.

6. Learning to live with limitations.

7. Learning about resources that can help.

8. Summary, evaluation and graduation.

Guest speakers will include physicians, nurses, social workers, nutritionists, physiotherapists, social security representatives, members of the clergy and representatives of the local cancer society and other community agencies. The I CAN COPE kit includes filmstrips, tapes and individual class outlines and this kit can be purchased from the American Cancer Society (for address see Appendix).

4.2.1.2. *The CanSurmont Programme*

This programme was initiated in June 1973 in Denver, Colorado, and exists to help people to a better understanding and coping with cancer. It is a volunteer programme which serves cancer patients, their families and those involved with the care and treatment of cancer patients. Because most CanSurmont volunteers have cancer themselves, they are in a position to add a unique dimension to the traditional health care team.

Patients need a special kind of support when living with, or dying from cancer and yet this need cannot always be satisfied by family, friends or professional personnel. The essential missing element is a shared experience with the person who has, or has had cancer himself and who is uniquely capable of better understanding the concerns, frustrations and fears of the patients. Should a cancer society establish a CanSurmont programme, the five basic activities will be:

1. To make patient visits on a regular basis.

2. To implement a visitation reporting system.

3. To keep the cancer society co-ordinator informed about activities.

4. To provide regular volunteer meetings.

5. To provide educational programmes for volunteers, patients and professionals.

The importance of proper selection and training for volunteers working in any CanSurmont programme cannot be over-emphasized. Such training will cover how to become effective listeners and communicators, discussion on individual reactions toward cancer and in-depth instructions on how to make good patient visitations. Further details from the American Cancer Society.

4.2.1.3. *'Candle lighters'*

In that sense of sharing problems and sorrows, association of parents of children with cancer have also been created in some countries.

The best known example of these are the 'Candle Lighters' which operate in the United States of America. The Candle Lighters are parents whose children have died from cancer, are long-term survivors or cured, or those whose children are still being treated. Formed originally to lobby for more funding of childhood cancer research, the Candle Lighter groups have gone on to many other activities such as monthly parents meetings with cancer professionals, periodic mutual support sessions, serving as second families, publication of news letters for and about their children, support for teenage cancer patients, social gatherings and fund raising projects.

4.2.2. *Programmes for Specific Patient Groups*

When the treatment of cancer involves extensive surgery, the problem of rehabilitation are so specific that special physical and/or psychological techniques are needed. Technical advances have been made in the rehabilitation of ostomy and laryngectomy patients and special teaching is part of the rehabilitation process. Mastectomy patients by the nature of their treatment undergo a physical trauma which provokes so many psychological reactions that very special readjustment is needed. Specific programmes have been developed to meet each of these needs and will be discussed in this section. However other groups of cancer patients may be numerically significant in different countries and in these cases the cancer society can develop rehabilitation programmes designed for their specific need.

4.2.2.1. *Mastectomy Patients*

In many cultures mastectomy is probably the most frightening operation that a woman can experience. She has to contend not only with a diagnosis of cancer, and with all the ancestral fears associated with it, but also with the fact that she has lost a very essential part of her feminine figure. Indeed many women look upon this operation as a terrible mutilation which provokes the fear of never being normal again. There is therefore always a depressive reaction in the early post-operative days with distressing concerns and anxiety about the attitudes of the sexual partner, the family and friends, but also worry about practical problems, like difficulties in finding the proper way to dress, the right prosthesis, etc.

In this difficult situation a woman who has herself had a mastectomy can provide invaluable assistance by showing the newly operated patient that it is possible not only to survive after a cancer operation, but also to live as a normal woman again. Various groups of volunteer mastectomy patients have come together throughout the world to help with the rehabilitation of their fellows. The best known of these is probably "The Reach To Recovery Programme" which started in America and has now spread throughout the world.

As the techniques and philosophy of the treatment for breast cancer are changing, with, in certain countries, a trend towards less radical surgery and even plastic breast implants, such mastectomy volunteer programmes have had to adapt and introduce

training of volunteers who have had implant surgery as well as
those who have had full mastectomy operations. In all cases,
however, the programmes operate with the approval of the attending
physician and with specially screened and trained volunteers who
visit the newly-operated woman in hospital, to assist her in her
physical, functional, psychological, emotional and social
rehabilitation. On a woman-to-woman basis, the volunteer will
give personal reassurance, assistance in the selection of prosthesis,
and provide helpful advice on other matters. A specially prepared
booklet may be available. In some countries a special lightweight
temporary prosthesis is provided to patients at this first visit.

Selection of Volunteers

The following criteria for the selection of volunteers will
be helpful to cancer societies considering the establishment of a
Mastectomy Advisory Service.

Firstly, a specified post-operative period should be stated
before a volunteer can be accepted for training. This will give
her time for physical and emotional adjustment after her own
treatment.

The cancer society co-ordinator of mastectomy services will
require all potential volunteers to complete an application form.
This will furnish information about the volunteer, her age, hobbies,
marital status, nature of operation and reasons for wanting to
become a volunteer helper. This form will usually be completed
prior to an interview with the co-ordinator, at which she can
assess the volunteer's personality and appearance etc, and general
suitability for the programme.

It is most important that volunteers should have a positive
attitude towards the medical and hospital services, and it is
essential that all volunteers must participate in a training
programme before being used.

Training of Mastectomy Volunteers

The following suggestions for training volunteers can be
adapted and modified for use by cancer societies. The same
programme could well be used for training cancer volunteers
involved in other types of rehabilitation programmes. It is
recommended that volunteers should attend six consecutive sessions
i.e. one per week for a six weekly period. Spreading out training
over this period enables the volunteer to absorb the information
and benefit fully from the discussion which takes place at training
sessions. It will also enable her to prepare for the next topic
to be discussed in training. Personnel likely to be involved in
training will be: the cancer society co-ordinator, surgeon, nurse,
a radiotherapist or oncologist, psychiatrist, and a trained
volunteer.

The co-ordinator will probably commence training sessions
with an over-view of the work of the mastectomy advisory programme
and of the cancer society in general. The American Cancer Society
"Reach to Recovery" film is a useful aid for the first training

session of volunteers. The co-ordinator will also describe
exactly what assistance they will be required to give during their
service with the programme. The description of prostheses and
special clothing used in the rehabilitation will also be given.

A senior nurse should speak about the organization of the
hospital ward, acquainting volunteers with the preparation and
aftercare of the patient following surgery. The surgeon will
give the history of cancer as a disease and a simplified
explanation of the various aspects of surgery. This would
include implantation of prostheses where this is current medical
practice.

A radiotherapist/oncologist will speak about radiotherapy
and adjuvant therapy and the psychiatrist will discuss the
psychological aspects of breast surgery and describe how patients
are counselled.

A trained volunteer, one who has had many years experience
in visiting patients can give useful, practical information to
the new volunteers and demonstrate how a visit should be carried
out. Each speaker in a training programme should have a
specialized knowledge of dealing with cancer patients. Throughout each session the importance of the volunteer not participating
in any medical counselling with patients is emphasized, as is the
importance of confidentiality and of being a good sympathetic
listener.

Hospital Visits by Volunteers

The best time to visit a mastectomy patient in hospital is
usually four to five days after her operation. The patient will
usually have been asked if she would like a visit from a volunteer.
Upon her consent a senior member of the hospital team involved
in the patient's care will normally contact the co-ordinator of
the cancer society giving details about the patient. At this
stage the co-ordinator will ask for some personal details
including her bust size in order that a temporary prosthesis may
be provided at this first visit. Upon receiving this information
the co-ordinator will contact a volunteer who will be most
suitable to this particular visit, i.e. try to match the age and
background of the patient as far as possible with that of the
visitor. The volunteer will herself then telephone the hospital
and make arrangements for a time suitable to both patient and
hospital for her visit. After the visit the volunteer will
forward a report to the co-ordinator.

Note: the same volunteer would normally visit this patient
again upon her return home from hospital.

In some countries a programme of pre-operative visits is also
organized. It is also possible to involve the husband as part of
the rehabilitation team.

4.2.2.2.   Laryngectomees

Laryngectomees have a very specific problem to overcome,
that of communication. To avoid the overwhelming fear that the

27

loss of voice will mean the inability to communicate with others
it is essential that the patient with the cancer of the larynx
who has had a laryngectomy performed should be informed before
operation of the possibilities of learning to speak and communicate
again with the oesophageal voice. Learning the oesophageal voice
is a very difficult task and it is important that team work
between the surgeon, nurses, speech therapist, social workers,
volunteers and the patients themselves, start before the operation
if success is to be achieved. Some hospitals may have a speech
therapy service. The local cancer society can provide funds for
the training of a speech therapist (where one does not exist),
by financing the purchase of special aids for laryngectomy
patients, and also through the creation, where necessary, of a
laryngectomy patients association. These associations have now
existed for many years in different countries and are usually
affiliated to the International Association of Laryngectomees.
Their help for laryngectomy patients is so important that it is
highly desirable that such an association exists in every country
where laryngeal cancer is a problem.

4.2.2.3. *Ostomy Patients*

In some cases of cancer of the bowel, as in some other
clinical situations, it is necessary for the surgeon to create
a new orifice (stoma) in the abdominal wall for the passage of
stools. This ileostomy or colostomy imposes completely different
ways of managing the movements of the bowels and this technique
has to be learned either in or outside the hospital. The same
radical change in the habits concern patients with a new opening
for the urine (urostomy) in place of the urinary bladder. Important
progress has now been made in the development of different
materials used for the stoma, such as self-adhesive plastic bags,
etc, and in the management of the stoma itself, so that it is
possible to bring about a complete rehabilitation to a normal life
for stoma patients. In some hospitals, specially trained nurses
(Stoma-therapists), are now used to care for ostomees and teach
them the best techniques.

Associations of ostomy patients have existed for several
years at both national and international level (International
Ostomy Association)† and cancer societies are often involved in
supporting them. Where these cancers are a problem a service of
ostomy volunteers, well adjusted to their surgery, may be
organized to visit newly operated patients with the approval of
the attending surgeon, offering useful help on a one-to-one
basis, and advising on a suitable diet. The availability of an
enterostomal therapist is also a concern of the cancer society which
can in certain instances provide financial support for training.

---

† *International Ostomy Association, 9135 Fordham Street,
Indianapolis, IN 46268, U S A*

4.2.2.4. *Other Specific Programmes*

Such programmes can be created every time volunteer patients can help their fellow-patients experiencing similar problems and difficulties. This might be after any severe surgery such as total gastrectomy, amputation of a leg or arm etc, but also after radiotherapy or chemotherapy. In all these cases, the patient-to-patient relation of the volunteer can be an invaluable help in rehabilitation.

4.3. *CARE OF THE DYING*

Despite the progress made in the management of cancer, people will continue to die of this disease. There is a natural fear of dying, but especially of dying from cancer, because of the general belief that this will always be associated with intractable pain. This is, of course, not true, not only because of progress made in the management of pain, but mainly because of the active interest of the medical oncology team in providing better help for the terminally ill patient. The concept of terminal care embraces all that is important for the well-being of the very ill, including the treatment of chronic pain. Despite the fact that this is a medical and even more a nursing problem, specially trained volunteers have a significant role to play in the team through visiting, providing companionship, comfort and recreation to patients.

4.3.1. *Domiciliary*

Very few people would choose to spend their final days in hospital where the activities in a busy ward are not conducive to coming to terms with death. Most people given the choice would wish to die at home close to family and friends. However, practical considerations often make it impossible to nurse patients adequately during this time. In certain areas, however, the cancer society can organize a special service for home health care, where specially trained volunteers would be a part of the team and would be a great help to the patient and his family.

4.3.2. *Special Hospital Units*

In an acute hospital the regime of care, the equipment etc, are all geared to treatment, cure and discharge and admission of the next patient on the waiting list. Staffing complements do not always allow for the individual attention and care needed to keep the dying person free from pain and discomfort and loneliness and to assist him and his family come to terms with approaching death.

The establishment of St Christopher's Hospice in London in 1968, gave impulse to the creation of special units where the terminally ill could receive all the care that they needed, more specifically the best possible palliation of pain and anxiety. There are some such special units around the world taking care of patients who are dying in the hospital, but very often these units also care for ambulatory patients, or even give domiciliary treatments.

This combination of in-patient, ambulatory and home care is the "Hospice Concept".

4.3.3.   *The Hospice Concept*

Hospice Treatment means care for a person according to his or her individual needs when curative or palliative treatment is no longer appropriate. Hospice care involves frequent very carefully monitored administration of drugs to allow the patient to remain mentally and physically alert and able, and in many cases, to enjoy a normal life while remaining free of pain. It involves taking a lot of time to identify causes of physical discomfort - breathlessness, nausea, etc, and to alleviate that distress. It also involves taking time to chat with a patient and his family, to answer their questions, to combat loneliness, to help them come to terms with death.

That is why hospices have been established in many countries. Hospices can provide four types of care:

- Home Care using a domiciliary team of doctors and nurses to assist the General Practitioner and the Community Nurse to care for the patient and support the family;

- Day Care by providing therapy etc in the hospice to home care patients who attend once or twice a week. They become familiar with the Hospice, get to know the staff, and the family at home are given a little respite;

- In-patient Care for those who have no-one to care for them at home or who have reached a stage in their illness where the family can no longer cope;

- Counselling and help to the family during the period of terminal illness and the bereavement period.

Hospices also aim to provide an educational service by teaching doctors pain control methods developed in hospices, by providing training appropriate to religious counsellors and social workers on the care of the terminally ill.

Two main types of hospice for the care of in-patients have been developed. Some are independent units, often sited in pleasant surroundings. Others are special hospice units attached to large general hospitals, where the hospice can share common services with the hospital.

The Hospice concept is a humane approach to medical care that deserves great support from the medical profession, hospital administration and local cancer societies, whose volunteers very carefully chosen and especially trained, are an important part of the programme. However, it should be noted that the establishment and maintenance of a hospice is a vastly expensive undertaking and cancer societies should ensure beforehand that any long-term commitment that they are going to make can be sustained and will not prejudice adequate support of other activities.

HELPFUL READING

Brugere, J., and Schraub, S. : Guide de reinsertion des cancereux
             traites. Doin, Editeur, Paris, 1980.

Kübler-Ross, Elisabeth : On Death and Dying. Tavistock Publications
             1970.

Markel, W.M., and Sinon, V.B. : The Hospice Concept. Ca 28. : 4,
             225-237. 1978.

Morris, T. : Psychological Adjustment to Mastectomy.
             Cancer Treatment Reviews, 6, 41-61, 1979.

Mount, B.M. : The Problem of Caring for the Dying in a General
             Hospital; the Palliative Care Unit as a
             Possible Solution.
             Canad. Med. Ass. J. 115, 119-121, 1976.

Domiciliary Care : Proceedings of a Seminar on Domiciliary Care.
             Abingdon, 1980. National Society for Cancer
             Relief. London.

Saunders, C. : The Need for In-patient Care for the Patient with
             Terminal Cancer.
             Middlesex Hosp. J., 72, 1973.

CHAPTER 5 - EDUCATION AND INFORMATION PROGRAMMES

INTRODUCTION

In every country in the world many more people could be cured of cancer if they were treated while their disease was more limited in its development. Others have cancers which could be prevented. In such cases the problem is not a failure of medical treatment, or of lack of knowledge how to prevent some cancers. It is rather a failure of patients or their doctors to take action soon enough. The problem therefore is one of human behaviour. To change behaviour implies education. The educational and informational activities of the cancer society, can, if effectively carried out, dramatically improve the prevention and the cure of cancers. Even where prevention or cure is not possible, early diagnosis can often do much to improve the patient's expectation and quality of life after treatment. Education also has an important part to play in other aspects of cancer control such as rehabilitation, after-care, and terminal care.

5.1. COMMITTEE STRUCTURE

To a large extent the image the cancer society presents to the community is formed by the quality and the nature of the informational and educational messages issued by the Education and Information Committee and it is therefore extremely important that its members should be selected with the greatest care. Their professional backgrounds should, if possible, reflect the wide range of training and experience that is needed to formulate a programme which has been designed on the basis of a complete understanding of the people it seeks to help. In this connection it should be realized that messages to the public proposed by the Fund-raising Committee should be harmonized with those of the Educational Committee. The committee structure of the Society in general should therefore be such as to ensure full collaboration between fund-raising and education so that apparently contradictory and confusing messages - "Help us to find a cure"; and "Cancer is curable" - are avoided. The size of the Committee on Education and Information will vary depending on circumstances, but if possible, the following disciplines and skills should be represented.

5.1.1. Doctors and Nurses

If the Society's message is to be respected by both the public and the medical profession it must be seen to have strong medical support. One or more clinicians experienced in the treatment of cancer are essential. However, eminent specialists are not always seen by generalist doctors to have an understanding of the difficulties which face those who have to deal every day with a wide range of sickness, both trivial and serious, and it may be wise to invite an experienced general practitioner to serve also. This member can gain the respect and support of his GP colleagues upon whose support and collaboration much of the success of the educational programme will depend. In addition, an epidemiologist, and/or a doctor concerned with public health, can

33

give valuable information about priority cancer health problems in the community. This is vital if the educational effort is to be directed towards the areas of greatest need, and if the programme is to be evaluated later. The medical members will see that statements to the public are medically accurate; they will keep the Society up-to-date with developments in research and treatment; and - very important - they will help the Society in its communications with doctors. Similarly the Committee will benefit from the services of senior nurses who can advise the Society and influence members of their profession.

5.1.2. *Educationists*

It is not enough that the Society should be supplied with accurate medical information. It should also benefit from the advice of committee members whose professional training fits them to understand how people learn and consequently what approaches may or may not be helpful. Such members should be able to take the medical facts and express them to the community in understandable and attractive terms, and in such ways as are more likely to change attitudes and behaviour. Because the processes of learning in adults are quite different from those in children it is desirable that both sections of the educational profession are represented. If the Society employs a full-time member of staff who is responsible to the Chief Executive for the public education programme this person should preferably have had professional training and experience in education.

He or she will work closely with the similarly-qualified volunteer committee members in planning both the content of the educational programme and the method by which it is to be addressed to the public. However, if the staff member has administrative rather than educational training it is vital to take seriously the advice of educationist committee members, on whose professional judgment the Society should rely implicitly. As in the practice of medicine, the planning and direction of education has little opportunity for amateurs however enthusiastic and imaginative they may be. It is also worth repeating here that opportunity should always be provided for the Education and Information Committee, and in particular its educationist members to comment on the educational implications of all the Society's communications to the general public.

5.1.3. *Social Scientists*

A sociologist - or a social psychologist - can give invaluable help in understanding the community; how people interact, what their normal pathways of communication are; their patterns of health behaviour and so on. This member, together with those trained in education, can also contribute significantly to research and evaluation in this area of the Society's activities.

5.1.4. *The Media*

The skills of journalists from newspapers and the broadcast media will be needed. Their roles are at least twofold. Firstly, although the Committee's business will be mainly education - which seeks to change attitudes and behaviour of individuals as well as to inform them - the information the Committee wishes to disseminate through the media must be accurate and not misleading so that it does not contradict educational objectives. Secondly, journalistic skills in helping to write the informational leaflets in simple, understandable terms are vital if much of the literature is not to prove a waste of time and money.

5.1.5.   Other Members

These should include community and religious leaders, social workers, and representatives of employers and workers. Commercial advertisers and publicists can make valuable contributions, but it is often wise to ensure, as with fund-raising messages, that their recommendations are not at variance with sound educational principles.

5.1.6.   Conclusion

The above represents a broad framework for a Committee on Education and Information showing the type of representation that is most desirable. If a University is near at hand, it can be very helpful to seek members from its academic staff. As well as bringing their expertise to the service of the Cancer Society in designing the programme, they may also be able to offer their students the possibility of educational and social research, the findings of which can monitor and evaluate the work. However, recruitment of volunteer committee members will clearly depend on national or local conditions.

5.1.7.   Checklist

- Does the Education and Information Committee represent all the skills and experience that are needed?

Clinicians experienced in cancer	Nursing	Sociology
General Medicine	Adult Education	Journalism
Epidemiology	Child Education	Community Workers
Public Health	Health Education	

- Has liaison been planned with other committees of the Society?

    Fundraising

    Patient Care

    Rehabilitation

    Terminal Care

5.2.   FACT-FINDING AND DATA COLLECTION FOR EDUCATION PROGRAMMES

What would be thought of a doctor who prescribed a treatment without listening to the patient's symptoms, without examining the patient beforehand, and without finding out about his later health? Careful preliminary data-collection - or periodic reviews of existing programmes - is just as important if an educational programme that meets the real needs of the community is to be prescribed. The more that is known before the educational planning stage the better.

5.2.1. Data Collection

Though this phase of the work need not be highly elaborate there are some areas of preliminary enquiry that are essential or near-essential. If people with the professional expertise and resources outlined in *5.1.* above have been attracted to the Committee the task will be easier. But if not, this should not necessarily be a reason for not trying to gather essential baseline information. It is of course assumed that the cancers are a significant health problem or that there is evidence they are about to become a problem.

5.2.1.1. Medical/Epidemiological

Some knowledge of the patterns of malignant disease in the population will be needed. What are the most common sites of cancer?

Which of these cancers are preventable? (e.g. lung cancer; cervix uteri; oral cancers; occupational cancers).

Which of these cancers are curable, and which cancers respond well to palliative treatment, given earlier diagnosis? Can we identify which sections of the population are most "at risk" for these diseases? (Are they: old/young; male/female; prosperous/disadvantaged; urban/rural; literate/illiterate; etc).

5.2.1.2. Medical Services

Are these adequate to meet any demand our message may create? (e.g. Pap smear; mammography; hospital facilities). If not should the Society's first priority be to help supply them? Or should the educational programme be promoted in the hope that pressure from the public may compel the authorities to improve services? But note that this form of action could mean a loss of the goodwill and the trust of a public who have responded to the message only to be disappointed by a lack of the service they have been promised. It may also produce hostility from the medical profession which may be made to appear inadequate or to feel pressurized by the cancer society.

5.2.1.3. The Public

To be effective all education of any kind <u>must</u> be based on an understanding of the learner's present position. In adults, both the ability and the willingness to learn is strongly influenced by what one already knows, and how one feels about the subject to be taught. When the subject is cancer most adults have "knowledge" of some kind. Even though this knowledge may be inaccurate (such as, for instance, the belief that all cancer is incurable) it must be remembered that this is reality for those who believe it, and that it is a reality which creates strong negative attitudes and therefore an unwillingness even to listen to messages about a subject that disturbs and frightens them.

In order to plan a programme that is suited to the needs of the community preliminary knowledge about the beliefs and attitudes that exist in different sections of society is essential. This

36

can be gathered in various ways, and will be greatly helped if committee members with special expertise have been chosen with care (see *5.1.* above). A traditional method is that of a study of public knowledge and opinion. For this the UICC Model Questionnaire may be adapted for local conditions. (See Appendix II, Page 113). There are, however, a number of important provisos if this method is used.

1. The questionnaire should be given to a properly-devised sample of the population so that the beliefs of different sections of society can be identified. This is best done by visiting a sample of people at home rather than in the street or market place.

2. If volunteers are used as interviewers they must have some training in interviewing techniques. For instance, they must not help respondents with their answers.

3. Careful analysis of the findings can show differences in knowledge and opinion among different sections of society. This will help in devising appropriate educational messages for each.

4. Periodic repeats of such a baseline study can monitor the programme by showing any changes in public knowledge and opinion.

However, other data can be collected that may influence the programme. Interested clinicians may be willing to investigate reasons for and causes of delay by patients. This may, for instance, show consistent patterns of fears, anxieties, and mistaken ideas about cancer and symptoms which the programme should seek to correct. And, for existing programmes that are in personal contact with the public, it can be very helpful for volunteers to record all questions addressed to them by the public over a defined period. In recording the questions that are important to individuals, areas of doubt and uncertainty in the public mind can be charted. This can illuminate the findings of other types of survey and also help refine and improve the educational programme.

Many cancer education workers complain that some groups are "hard to reach" even though these are often the most in need of the educational message. However, this is in fact most often the fault of the educator, who has failed to find out about those he wishes to educate. Some preliminary studies can reduce this problem.

It is important to understand the networks of communication that exist in sub-sections of society, and especially those that are identified as high-risk or target groups. They may be hard to reach because they are geographically at a distance from the Society's office; because there are ethnic or language differences; because, since they live in rural communities, they have different perceptions from city-dwellers about how sickness is defined and when one should consult the doctor; because they fear cancer above all else and are therefore deaf to messages about the disease; because they are either illiterate or functionally illiterate, and so on.

In many cases it may be possible to identify local community leaders through whose co-operation the message may be channelled. They may be persons elected to office, or they may simply be individuals with no formal position but to whom everyone turns for help and advice. These may sometimes be identified simply by asking all individuals to name someone in a local community they admire and respect. Often one or two names emerge as being most frequently mentioned.

It may also help to enquire about other health-related programmes in the past, and to try to identify the reasons for success or failure. There may be the possibility of joining forces with other health education workers in the community.

5.2.1.4. Health Professionals

The collaboration of doctors, nurses and paramedical workers is vital. The cancer society may want to know what are their attitudes to cancer, and to the idea of public education about cancer. Such enquiries will often reveal a need for <u>professional</u> education in cancer. Enquiries in this field are best conducted by medical and other appropriate professional persons.

5.2.1.5. Checklist

- *What are the main cancer problems? Which can be tackled by changing behaviour?*

- *Check medical services. Are they adequate?*

- *What does the public know about the cancers? What are their attitudes?*

- *What sections of the public are hard to reach? Why?*

- *What can we learn from other health education programmes? Can we collaborate with them?*

- *What do doctors and nurses know and feel about cancer? Is there a need for professional education?*

5.3. PLANNING EDUCATIONAL PROGRAMMES

5.3.1. General Principles

Having collected data that charts the community - its patterns of cancer, its medical services, its geographical and social characteristics, the level of knowledge and the attitudes of sub-sections of society to malignant diseases - the educational effort can now be planned. On the basis of fact-finding, certain disease priorities may have emerged, such as cervical cancer, lung cancer, and so on. But if the Committee wishes individuals to act with a clear understanding of the implications of what they are doing, it is most desirable to make sure people have a balanced picture of the cancers in general. Among other things this implies an understanding of a group of related, non-infectious diseases, of which some are preventable, some incurable, some normally difficult to diagnose at an early stage, many highly curable with early diagnosis and treatment, and most more easily controlled when treated early rather than late. Given this background information people find it more easy to accept education about cancers in specific sites.

However, in the context of cancer education "the general
public" as a concept simply does not exist. Having gone some way
to identifying "high risk" groups, and having also identified
different sections of society with different levels of literacy,
life-styles, values and so on it is clearly impossible to plan
any one message that would be understood by the whole population.
This calls for the development of different educational
prescriptions for the different sections of society such as are
outlined in section *5.4.1.* which follows. In each case it is
profitable to begin by asking the questions "what do we wish these
people to know?" and "what do we wish them to do?" This leads
logically to the task of defining specific and measurable
educational objectives. For instance the statement "After our
programme women will be more aware of the Pap smear service" is
unsatisfactory because "more aware" is not measurable. But
objectives such as "After the programme a woman will be able to
select correctly from a list of choices the purpose of the Pap
smear; state where it is available; state when she last had one
taken, and when she should attend for the next" are precise and
testable objectives that are measurable in educational and
behavioural terms.

5.3.2.   *Educational Programme Content*

The desirability of helping people to develop a balanced
view of the cancers has already been mentioned. In most countries
where they have been carried out, studies have shown that fear of
cancer as well as ignorance of symptoms is a cause of delay in
seeking medical advice or participating in cancer screening. If
fear is a cause of delay, adding to these fears is not likely to
make people behave differently, and indeed most research into the
effects of fear-arousing education has shown it to be ineffective
or even harmful. Therefore, all messages should, where justifiable,
have a reassuring content. But the message must be truthful. If
members of the public believe they have discovered untruths in
statements made by the Cancer Society they may justifiably suspect
everything that is said, with serious effects on the educational
work. Thus the statement "With early treatment cancer of the
cervix is curable in most cases" is true; whereas "With early
treatment all cancer is curable" is not true. Symptoms might best
be described as warning signs of ill-health of which cancer is
often the least likely explanation. This is truthful, and may be
of help to patients who would tend to delay having symptoms
investigated if they thought cancer to be the only, or the most
frequent explanation. It may be possible also to devise a message
describing positive steps people can take to guard their own
health; "Have a regular health check; Have a Pap smear; Examine
your breasts; Don't smoke" and so on. But if such messages are
planned it is vital to make sure beforehand that the services
advertised are adequate to meet the potential demand. Within
these general guidelines education about cancers in specific sites,
according to the priorities already identified, may be planned.
In addition, many communities need strong and sustained warnings
about unorthodox practitioners and unproven methods of treatment.
As representing orthodox medical opinion on established and proven
methods, the Cancer Society has an important role in exposing
fraudulent claims and teaching the public to look critically at

pseudo-scientific literature which purports to "prove" the
effectiveness of various treatments.

5.3.3. *Educational Programme Methodology*

Where the need is to change attitudes and behaviour, there
is no adequate substitute for person-to-person methods of education,
especially where individuals are given the opportunity to ask
questions that are important to them. This is the most effective
way of correcting mistaken ideas and eradicating the needless fears
that arise from misconceptions and superstitions. To provide such
a service implies recruiting volunteers - preferably doctors or other
health professionals who know the subject - who will visit and
give talks to groups in the community. However, such personnel
are not usually trained in educational techniques and it may be
desirable to arrange briefing sessions - with the help of
appropriate Committee members or others - in the use of visual
aids and in developing the skills necessary to conduct dialogues
with groups of different educational backgrounds and levels of
understanding. Another important factor in recruiting people to
speak to the public is that such volunteers - and members and
staff of the Cancer Society too - should be non-smokers.

Visual aids are important, but are not a substitute for
discussion and question-and-answer. Many visual aids are in use
in many countries and their suitability should be reviewed.
However, it is seldom the case that visual aids transfer easily
from one country to another, or from one culture to another
within the same country; where the resources are available it may
be preferable to make new ones suited to local conditions, perhaps
using ideas from other organizations, but revised to suit the
local populations we wish to educate. (See UICC Compilation of
Audio-Visual Resources listed in references on page 48.)

Given a programme based on personal methods the mass media
can provide valuable reinforcement provided that apparently-
contradictory statements are avoided. This is true of all broadcast media. As for printed material, leaflets in particular have
been shown to have great value when handed to individuals who have
just heard a talk on the subject. As with visual aids, it is
seldom the case that leaflets from one country or culture can be
used without modification elsewhere. If in doubt, there are
guidelines that can be used for testing the readability and value
of printed matter. It may be necessary to devise different
leaflets on the same topic for different sections of the population.

5.3.4. *Checklist*

- *What are the social and psychological characteristics of target groups?
  What do we wish them to know? To do?*

- *Have we defined learning objectives for each target group? In general,
  what is to be the content of the education programme?*

- *Do our findings so far show how the education is to be mediated? (Person-
  to-person; mass media; a combination of both?)*

- *If person-to-person, who is to do the educating? (Doctors, nurses, Society
  staff, etc).*

- *Do they need training in educational techniques?*

- *What visual aids, leaflets, posters are available? Are they really
  suitable? Do we need to make our own? Have we tested them among groups
  they are intended for?*

5.4. IMPLEMENTING THE EDUCATIONAL PROGRAMME

5.4.1. Tell the Doctors

After the general programme has been planned a first vital
step is to talk to the medical profession. Every practising
clinician should know precisely what is being proposed and what the
aims and objectives are. This has at least two advantages. In
providing doctors with the opportunity to offer advice to the
Cancer Society and satisfy themselves that no psychological harm
is likely to be done to their future patients, it creates a fund
of goodwill beneficial to the Cancer Society. And another, more
subtle advantage is that it may make some general practitioners
more alert to the possibility of a diagnosis of cancer in patients
who consult them. Both here, and in the matter of professional
education, the initiatives should be taken by medical members of
the Cancer Society.

5.4.2. Community Groups

In most communities people get together in groups for a
number of reasons - religious, social and political. An index of
such groups, will provide a rich source for talks on cancer. A
letter addressed personally to the group secretary or organizer
describing the lecture service and offering a speaker, is more
likely to gain a response than one that is impersonal. One talk
to a given group is not enough, and planning should cater for
repeat, periodic visits to each group. This will necessitate
different visual aids, and perhaps different topics so that groups
receive a programme of talks over a period of years each building
on information given on the first, general talk on the cancers.

5.4.3. Schools

If the problem of fears arising from public superstitions
and misconceptions are not to be perpetuated from one generation
to the next, children must be protected by suitable education about
cancer. Though the methods of doing this may differ from one
country to another, it is probably best to ensure that this is
done by the children's own teachers in the normal course of subject
teaching in class. Teachers themselves are much more likely to
respond positively if they are provided with materials they can
use rather than to moral exhortations that they should do something
about cancer. A number of countries have successfully translated
the UICC's 'Cancer Education in Schools - A Guidebook For Teachers'
into their own languages for the use of biology teachers. In
addition, materials for teachers and students, covering a wider
range of curriculum subjects, are in use in some countries. First
approaches to teachers are best made through educational members
of the Committee. The UICC organizes regional workshops on Cancer
Education in Schools to help Cancer Societies in this field.

5.4.4. Employee Groups

Many individuals, who do not attend meetings of community groups, may be reached where they work. Programmes addressed to workers should be suited to local conditions. The ideal is probably to arrange talks to workpeople followed by questions. Strategies to arrange such talks are most likely to succeed if they include approaches to both management and workers' representatives. To reinforce personal methods of education, or, as a substitute if other approaches fail, it may be possible to include suitable literature in pay packets.

5.4.5. Doctors and Nursing

The education of doctors and nurses has a dual role. First it can draw attention to the educational needs of the public and to the informal role of many professionals in responding to questions about cancer from relatives and friends. In this connection it may be possible through professional Committee members to arrange lectures to medical, nursing and other students. However, it should be borne in mind that professionals in general are trained to form opinions on the basis of evidence rather than to appeal to some moral obligation. The Society's case will be considerably strengthened if it has data to present which are based on studies of public opinion and patient behaviour in relation to cancer.

Doctors, and especially those in general practice, have a profound influence on the behaviour of their patients. UICC has evolved a strategy for involving doctors in health education about cancer. (See References for UICC Technical Report on Doctor Involvement in Public Education about Cancer). The second role of professional education lies in ensuring that clinical teaching of students about cancer is up-to-date and has an adequate place in the medical and nursing curriculum. This is a matter for discussion with those responsible for professional training and should be the exclusive responsibility of professionals serving on the Committee.

Medical and nursing professionals in many countries still regard the activities of cancer leagues and societies with suspicion and do not favour public education about cancer. Often this is due to a failure of the Cancer Society to communicate with doctors and nurses often enough, or in terms that appeal to their professional viewpoints. One means of overcoming objections and setting up more cordial and understanding relationships is for professional members of the Committee to ensure that medical and nursing meetings and conferences give opportunity for lectures on the public educational implications of the particular disease problems that are being discussed.

5.4.6. Other Caring Groups

Other professionals, such as radiographers, responsible for operating X-ray therapy machinery; hospital physicists, physiotherapists, social workers, all have an important educative function. So also have doctors' secretaries, ancillary hospital staffs, and many others working in the health and community welfare

fields. None should be omitted in ensuring that all individuals
whose advice may be sought are thoroughly briefed in the need for
informed and sensitive education of members of the public.

5.4.7.   Checklist

- *Have we discussed our intentions and plans beforehand with the medical profession? Who else should know what we propose?*

- *What do we know about our communities? What groups exist? Who are the community leaders?*

- *What plans have we for schools? What materials do we need? How can we get teachers to collaborate?*

- *What plans have we to reach people at work?*

- *What about professional education to alert doctors and nurses as to their informal role as educators of relatives and friends? What other health workers should we contact?*

5.5.   MONITORING AND EVALUATING EDUCATIONAL PROGRAMMES

If education is capable of changing people's attitudes and
behaviour it is also true that, like many pharmaceutical products,
it may have undesirable side-effects.

5.5.1.   Importance of Evaluation

Evaluating the effects of the educational work is therefore
important not only so that the work may be refined and improved
but also so that any approaches which may be doing harm may be
detected and eliminated. For instance enquiries into the attitudes
and knowledge of schoolchildren about cancer have revealed that
previous attempts to discourage them from smoking by an undue
emphasis on the threat and nature of lung cancer had produced in
them a distorted and potentially harmful view of the cancers in
general. This, incidentally, is a further indication that it is
unwise to restrict cancer education to one site of the disease.
Responsible health education about cancer will therefore always
include some measurement of results. Large-scale studies, though
very useful for some purposes, are costly. But if finance is
limited, small-scale enquiries should be within the capabilities
of every cancer society. This section briefly outlines some
possibilities.

5.5.2.   Public Opinion Surveys

As discussed above (5.2.1.3.) a well-designed survey of public
opinion can give a good indication of the levels of knowledge of
various sections of the community and some idea of possible
attitudes. If such a base-line survey is done, this can be
repeated periodically to check whether public knowledge is
changing. Repeat studies should, of course, be conducted in the
same population for purposes of comparison, but random selection
of those to be interviewed should be on a different basis so that
the same individuals are not interviewed again. A further
refinement of this method would be to find a control population
which will not receive education for the time being, and which is

matched as closely as possible with the population to be educated. Later comparisons might then be made between the educated and non-educated communities.

Such studies are best suited to revealing what people actually know, and to a much lesser extent their attitudes and behaviour. Because one aim of the educational programme will be to increase accurate knowledge on crucial points (for instance the knowledge that cancer is sometimes or often curable; and that early treatment makes a difference) this is a useful instrument for such measurements. But see also 5.5.4. below.

5.5.3.   *Studies of behaviour change*

Response to some messages will take the form of action on the individual's part. Some studies of action, like reported reduction in smoking, or statements about breast self-examination, are less reliable because there is no easy way of verifying that what the individual says is true. However, other behaviour can be measured accurately, such as counting how many women have requested a Pap smear. But in such cases, accurate record-taking is very important. It is easy to be misled into believing a Pap-smear programme, for instance, has been highly successful simply because of a response from large numbers of women. The real question is not how many women responded, but what proportion of women in high-risk categories have done so. Only by recording information about those who respond, such as age, marital status, parity, husband's occupation, place of residence etc, can some impression be gained whether the programme has been really effective in reaching at-risk persons.

If aims and objectives have been clearly defined one important, but difficult question to answer is how many more patients with malignant disease have reported symptoms to the doctor promptly. If hospital records are adequate these should show trends over a period of time. But in effect the true measurement of such actions is to be found in the offices of general practitioners, for most of the patients who responded by consulting the doctor will not in fact have cancer. It may be possible to gain the co-operation of local doctors in recording the number of patients who report given symptoms promptly - say post-menopausal or rectal bleeding - before and after some special educational effort.

5.5.4.   *Studies within the Educational Programme*

A useful way of gaining insights into public concerns and uncertainties about cancer is to listen to their questions. If a service of talks on cancer is in operation, volunteer speakers can be asked to co-operate by recording questions asked during discussion-time. A check-list for speakers is helpful. Given that sufficient numbers are collected, and that they cover an adequate cross-section of groups in the community, collation and analysis of these data can be most revealing and can help modify programme content. An analysis of written and verbal enquiries to the cancer society also provides useful data. These help illuminate the findings of public opinion surveys but should be seen as complementary rather than as a substitute for them.

The cancer society should also have a clear idea whether given talks or the visual aids that illustrate them, are helpful and understood. Indeed, all new visual aids should be tested before they come into general use. If educational objectives have been clearly stated beforehand "What do we want people to know?" (see 5.3.1. above) members of the groups can be asked to complete short questionnaires to elucidate what they have learned. In such cases it is often useful to ask the question indirectly: questions such as "Have you learned anything you did not know before?" may produce a majority of negative answers; whereas questions like "Do you think .... is not generally known?" may produce much fuller responses. People do not like to admit to ignorance themselves.

5.5.5.   *Checklist*

- *How are we to evaluate the programme in the long term? What evidence shall we seek? (Changes in knowledge; in behaviour of patients).*

- *Has short-term monitoring been arranged? (Questions from public: evaluation of visual aids, etc).*

5.6.   *FINANCING AN EDUCATION AND INFORMATION PROGRAMME*

Public knowledge and attitudes, and the behaviour of patients, do not change quickly, however enlightened and intensive the educational programme may be. The problem calls for long and sustained effort over many years, and an attitude of mind that sees temporary discouragements as opportunities for constant revision and refinements of educational techniques.

Financial planning - of every stage and aspect of the programme - should reflect an awareness that this will be the case. Because it is better from an educational point of view to plan a programme into which education about particular cancers is set in the context of education about the cancers as a whole, societies with limited funds may be wise to begin with small, but complete programmes in selected localities rather than to attempt ambitious efforts to reach the whole population at once.

It should be remembered that education which is effective and acceptable to the professions and the public is likely to attract more voluntary giving, some of which can be ploughed back into the educational work and so promote a gradual and healthy growth of the activity.

5.6.1.   *Checklist*

- *Has finance been arranged in advance of every stage. Plans should be for long term.*

5.7.   *EDUCATION AND INFORMATION IN THE CONTEXT OF CANCER CONTROL*

A national or regional programme of cancer control should pay attention to: 1) Prevention; 2) Screening; 3) Early diagnosis; 4) Treatment; 5) Patient care and after-care; 6) Rehabilitation; and 7) Terminal care. Education and information play a vital part in all of these activities, and education of the public is implied especially in 1, 2, 3, 5 and 6 above. If the Cancer Society's role in any of them is to be respected by the professions and to be of most value to the public, it should be carried out with the same care and professionalism that is shown in the medical treatment of patients.

This section on Education and Information has given broad guidelines on how this might be achieved. Financial or other constraints may limit the extent to which individual cancer organizations can follow all of the recommendations made, but some, which are not expensive, are well within the capabilities of most Societies. It is really a matter of adopting an attitude of mind that critically examines existing work and proposals for new ventures, and does not mistake effort for achievement. Enthusiasm alone is not enough if we are to solve the complex and difficult problems of changing attitudes and behaviour - both professional and public - in relation to cancer. If the Education and Information Committee has been selected with care, and all its members are persuaded of the desirability of such an approach to the task this will inevitably influence both the content of public education and the methods by which it is carried out, and will result in a programme most likely to be respected and, above all, effective in helping to save lives.

HELPFUL READING

UICC Publications
Union International Contre le Cancer
3 rue du Conseil-General, 1205 Geneva, Switzerland

Over the years UICC has produced many Technical Reports under the general heading Public Education About Cancer. They contain papers by experienced authors on all aspects of cancer education of the public, and reflect a high degree of professionalism. Heavy demand has depleted stocks of some earlier publications, but the publications listed below are currently available. The Geneva office will be happy to help members who are seeking information on aspects of public education and to advise which publications are available in languages other than English.

Public Education About Cancer. UICC Technical Report Series.

Vol 26 (1977) Includes : Smoking habits and attitudes; attitudes to breast cancer; response to screening programmes; opinions of schoolchildren about cancer; public education programmes; attitudes of cancer patients; doctors as educators; educating medical students.

Vol 31 (1978) Includes : The mass media and cancer; community education, and education in the workplace; smoking and health; education and screening for breast, cervical, and colo-rectal cancer; smoking and health professionals.

Vol 45 (1979) Includes : Community responsibilities in prevention and control; schoolchildren's attitudes, and development and evaluation of multidisciplinary resource package for schools; preventing onset of smoking, and fight against nicotine addiction; newspaper coverage of cancer; knowledge of, and participation in screening and cancer tests; industrial cancer education.

Vol 55 (1980) Includes : Health education about pre-cancerous lesions; community programmes on breast and cervical cancer and their effectiveness; worry related to teaching BSE; public use of cancer information service; designing educational leaflets.

Vol 62 (1981) Includes : conceptions, misconceptions, and perceptions of various groups about aspects of cancer; food habits; readership of BSE leaflets; participation in cervical screening.

Vol 67 (1982) Includes : Psychological problems in screening; psychology of communication; rural and Asian cancer communication and education; knowledge of cancer among schoolchildren; evaluation of stop-smoking methods; BSE and further information demanded by women being taught it.

Doctors as educators

Vol 44 (1979) Involving Doctors in Health Education about Cancer.
This monograph to guide health education planners wishing to
involve doctors in public education programmes describes useful
strategies and tactics that may be adapted to fit local conditions.
A very valuable handbook for all health educators who wish to gain
the respect and collaboration of physicians.

Smoking

Vol 28 (1977) Lung Cancer Prevention : Guidebook for Smoking Control.
A handbook dealing comprehensively with how the smoking problem
should be tackled via political, social and educational strategies.

Vol 52 (1980) A second edition of the above, based on the findings
of many Workshops arising from Vol 28. (Also published in Spanish).

Visual Aids

Vol 46 (1979) Slide Compilation of Cancer Control Posters.
Describes availability of colour-slide reproductions of cancer
posters from many countries, many of which might be adapted by
Leagues and Societies for their own use.

Vol 29 (1977) International Catalogue of Films, Filmstrips and
Slides on Public Education About Cancer.
A wide-ranging list of audio/visual materials from many countries.
In English, French, and Spanish.

Vol 54 (1980) First supplement to the above.

Schools Education

Vol 38 (1978) Cancer Education in Schools : A Guidebook for
Teachers.
A biology-based guidebo6k designed to fit various parts of the
school curriculum. Contains seven lessons, each divided into
scven sections. Sections cover a comprehensive learning
experience in distinct steps from the information students need
before each lesson, to final evaluation. This has now been
translated into many languages.

OTHER PUBLICATIONS

Pre-testing in Health Communications. US Department of Health and
Human Services. National Institutes of Health. Washington DC,
USA. A useful guide to testing the comprehensibility of printed
health messages.

Persons at High Risk of Cancer : An approach to Cancer Etiology
and Control. Ed. Fraumeni, Joseph F Jnr (1975). Academic Press.
New York. A guide to identifying persons in special need of
education for cancer prevention.

Cancer Campaign. Chapter in Cancer Control Vol II. Ed. Smith
and Alvarez. (1979) Pages 61 - 115. Pergamon Press. London

and New York. Contains many useful papers on public cancer
education presented at the 12th International Cancer Congress,
Buenos Aires. 1978.

Understanding Cancer : a guide for the caring professions (1977)
Ed. Burn and Meyrick. Her Majesty's Stationery Office, London.
A very readable book aimed at informing all professionals involved
in caring for patients, and in pointing to their role as educators.

Unproven Methods of Cancer Management. American Cancer Society Inc.
777 Third Avenue, New York, NY 10017. A useful guide for all
Leagues and Societies who meet problems of unorthodox practitioners
in the community. As well as exposing the characteristic devices
employed by quacks to deceive the public, it also describes how
various unorthodox treatments have been tested scientifically and
found to be ineffective.

EDUCATING SCHOOLCHILDREN

As well as the UICC's Guidebook for Teachers (see above) a number
of individual Societies have produced materials for use in Schools.
Many show a high degree of imagination and professional excellence,
and adaptations of them might usefully supplement the UICC
publication Vol 38. They are too numerous to describe here, but
a list of organizations to which one might apply are shown as an
Appendix to Vol 38 (see above).

CHAPTER 6 - SMOKING CONTROL ACTIVITIES

INTRODUCTION

Smoking is a widespread and universal habit. In some of the industrialised countries the rate of smoking is decreasing; in many developing countries it is now starting to rise.

Cancer is a problem in every country. Much effort is needed to clarify the roles of the various carcinogens and cancer mechanisms. Paradoxically those cancers of which the causes are best understood and preventable seem in fact to be the very cancers that are increasing. A second paradox is that although smoking is one of the greatest avoidable health hazards of modern times, much more effort is given to other health problems. Many countries have gone through a painful trial-and-error procedure in first allowing and later trying to hinder the spreading of this priority health hazard. Much can be done before the problem gets out of hand.

At first, smoking was used mostly to increase the enjoyment of life. The tobacco industry has always supported this idea. Smokers do look happy and healthy in tobacco advertisements. But a third paradox is that smoking calms or reassures only the smoker. For a non-smoker a cigarette gives no pleasure. And regular smokers are less healthy than non-smokers. Many investigations prove that even a young smoker experiences a wide range of symptoms and does not feel healthy.

It is also well-known that the reasons for starting to smoke differ from the motivation to continue smoking. A youngster starts to smoke from curiosity, peer influence and availability of cigarettes. Later on he or she may become dependent on smoking. A great majority of smokers want to stop smoking and many try this often. In the case of nations the reasons for allowing smoking to become a habit in society may also differ from the reasons to continue. Many complicated economic pressures may make a country dependent on tobacco imports, industry or cultivation.

Smoking has economic implications. At first sight it may seem that the taxation revenues are so great that smoking is economically beneficial for a country. But this is not so. Costs for excess mortality and morbidity as well as other losses due to smoking exceed the revenues it confers.[1] Fifty eight percent of tobacco is grown in the developing countries, but the benefits for this are not stationary. Tobacco uses the same land which could bring more important products. Because its cultivation is seasonal, workers are unemployed for many months of the year. This applies especially to small farms. Tobacco may also cause import/export balance disturbances.

6.1.1.   The Role of the Cancer Society

In countries where smoking has been a widespread habit it is responsible for 90 percent of deaths from lung cancer, for 75 percent of deaths from bronchitis, and for 25 percent of deaths from ischaemic heart disease among men under 65 years of age. In women these proportions may be somewhat lower depending on the fact that smoking has not spread equally among both sexes. It has also been estimated that without smoking the total cancer death rate would be reduced by a quarter.

Despite this indisputable and mounting evidence of the health hazards of smoking the growth, manufacture and use of tobacco are increasing in the world. It has been said that the smoking habit spreads like an epidemic. The increase of death and disease will continue unless the increase in cigarette consumption is reversed. No greater challenge faces cancer societies than the control of the several cancers related to smoking.

The role of a Cancer Society depends on the national situation regarding smoking. Where smoking is already common the strategies to reduce it differ from those to halt or reverse the growth of the smoking habit. There are, however, pre-requisites applicable to all countries whatever their smoking history has been.

There is no single measure to solve the problem on its own. A comprehensive programme is essential. The programme should be constructive, emphasising the positive effects of remaining a non-smoker. The programme should not attack smokers too strongly or arouse fear. Its basis should be medically strong and the emphasis should lie on health policy aspects.

Cancer societies can collect and spread information on different components of the programme. They can plan and promote health education; act as opinion leaders to foster a positive attitude towards a smoke-free society. Cancer societies can exert strong pressure in matters of legislation, and also on the mass media.

A society can bring together expertise in medicine, jurisprudence, social sciences, psychology, education, public health, mass media etc to provide a balanced and modern approach. It may also promote and provide funds for such a comprehensive anti-smoking programme. International co-operation is helpful.

The tobacco industry is responsible for spreading the smoking epidemic. Local tobacco cultivators cannot be blamed for this. But cancer societies can give all support to governments in their efforts to implement the WHO recommendations approved by the governments of WHO members. According to these recommendations tobacco export, cultivation and industry is to be limited and sales promotion prohibited everywhere in the world.

6.1.2.   *Overall Strategies for Smoking Control*

A smoking control programme needs clear and well-defined objectives, sound basis, good co-operation, adequate resources, and sound evaluation. These are the general policy objectives of the UICC in its endeavour to stimulate international control of smoking. The UICC is concerned primarily with cigarette smoking as the avoidable cause of most lung cancer, but its recommendations have obvious relevance to other smoking-associated cancers and other diseases also caused partly or wholly by smoking.

These objectives have been adopted by WHO[2] and are suitable bases for an international approach to control of one of the most important disease groups afflicting twentieth century society.

1. Achievement of lower smoking rates in all age-groups of the population. This implies the application of whatever downward pressures on smoking rates that are practical. These might include health warnings on packets, taxation manipulation, restrictions on smoking opportunities, encouragement of the rights of the non-smoker, as well as measures such as are involved in political, publicity and education programmes.

2. The encouragement of non-smokers to remain non-smokers. The emphasis of this programme is on youth.

3. The cessation of all forms of tobacco promotion.

4. Those who have not yet stopped smoking, and therefore remain at high risk, should be encouraged to reduce, as far as possible, their exposure to harmful components of tobacco smoke.

5. To maintain liaison with other health organizations and authorities to ensure maximum effectiveness and avoid conflict of activities.

6. To achieve public health control of relevant industrial and environmental factors which contribute to lung cancer.

No matter how vigorous an effort is, little is achieved if the message is unclear, unreliable or is not accepted by other health agencies or health officials. Co-operation is essential. The message to the public needs support from every group concerned. Much more will be learned if the programme is carefully evaluated both during and after the project. The need for evaluation and documentation should be taken into account when estimating the resources needed.

The ultimate objective of the programme is obviously to decrease smoking-related diseases. For this it is necessary[3]:

- to change the behaviour of the smoker and to maintain that of the non-smoker

- to change the cultural background of society against which cigarette smoking is often viewed as a status symbol representing success and sophistication; to establish the realistic view which is that cigarettes are both unnecessary and hazardous

- to change the economic and legislative climate so that cigarettes are less readily available; that pressures promoting smoking are ceased and education programmes are supported and reinforced

- to change the cigarette smoked so that it is less harmful

- to establish non-smoking as the norm, and to ensure the right of the non-smoker to clean air

The possible components of the programme are:

- a suitable economic and social analysis of the local smoking problem

- a public information programme

- public education programmes aimed at adults, exemplar groups, adolescents, and children. Within this programme special projects are needed to help committed smokers who have particularly high risk, such as pregnant women, asbestos workers, and so on

- a legislative programme

- access to schools, the media, and help from other agencies to deliver programmes once developed

The smoker is not always conscious of running into danger but may ignore the risk or consider it to be remote and rather improbable. Yet the evidence is indisputable and conclusive. The first scientific report on the relations of smoking and lung cancer was published as early as 1761[4]. The evidence of involuntary (passive) smoking as a cause of lung cancer was presented in 1981[5,6]. In between, several other effects have been documented many of which are seriously disabling and irreversible. It even seems that the more serious the disease is, the later the symptoms appear. This may in part explain why the smoker who has at the moment no distinct symptoms does not feel himself to be particularly more "at risk".

Information on the harmfulness of smoking must therefore be passed to the public.

Nations differ from each other in how well-informed their citizens are in these matters. In many developed countries facts concerning the health consequences of smoking have reached the public; but in others, people are almost unaware of these consequences. In the latter case it is crucial to ensure that the health message reaches all sectors of society (field workers, physicians, decision makers etc) and not solely the public in general. The message must be delivered to all whose activities can support it. However, it should be remembered that even where the health risks are widely known, smokers tend not to accept that they themselves are highly at risk.

A co-ordinating group, where government and non-government bodies are represented is needed when planning a comprehensive smoking control programme and choosing priorities, target groups, methods and overall policy. The Cancer Society also needs a smoking control group of its own, which may be a part of the Education and Information Committee.

Realism is needed when plans are made for overall strategies and objectives. If too much is expected and too little time and resources are available, poor results can disappoint and discourage. Changes in the opinion climate, and in legislation and in health behaviour happen very slowly. The chain reaction from knowledge to attitudes and from attitudes to behaviour is not quick; neither does it always happen in this order.

The objective is not to create an atmosphere when people eagerly change from one health habit to another depending on the sender of the most recent message (e.g. Tobacco industry or a Cancer Society). The aim is rather to help people to become aware of the overall consequences of health behaviour and self-care. To achieve this may be slow. Health education experts are needed to provide for continuous and reliable health education. These people work on a long-term basis, which ensures also evaluation, documenting and publishing of results. Active and enthusiastic volunteers, such as opinion leaders and those who can exert social and political pressure, are indeed an essential part of a smoking control programme. But a comprehensive and effective smoking-reducing programme needs a continuity which is best ensured by a permanent committee and staff.

Zero or negative results of programmes or campaigns in many fields of activity and in many countries are unfortunately seldom published. Expectations may therefore be too high when initiating the smoking control programme. Information from other countries about similar smoking control programmes may help in planning, but a programme which has been effective in one country or culture may not function elsewhere. More is needed than translation. Overall strategies of a smoking control policy are tightly bound with the national and local situation.

6.1.3. *Public Information Programmes*

Public information is an important part of a comprehensive smoking control programme. Smoking touches almost every individual. Current smokers have approximately 70 percent greater chance of dying within a specific age span than non-smokers. Ex-smokers experience declining mortality ratios as the years of cessation increase[2]. It has been estimated, that in Britain, 30 - 50 percent of smokers die because of their smoking[7]. Female smokers experience mortality ratios similar to those of male smokers. Smoking affects those who surround the smokers at home[5,6] and at the workplace. Smoking also affects recovery from operations[8] and seems even to facilitate the spread of metastases in some cancers [9,10]. It has also been found out that continuation of smoking during the treatment of small cell lung cancer is associated with a poor prognosis while discontinuation of smoking, even at diagnosis, may have beneficial effects on survival[11]. Smoking has implications other than those connected to cancers.

Smoking therefore affects the whole population in countries where active smoking is common. Some of the smokers are involuntary (passive). The more the health consequences of smoking are investigated the more-faceted the picture becomes. It concerns the healthy public; those at risk; and even the patients who already have cancer. The message must, therefore, be tailored differently for various groups of people and this is what makes a reliance on mass media alone unrealistic. There is no one mass message that is helpful to all. And in any case a clear distinction should be made between the dissemination of information via the media, and face-to-face eduation, which is more appropriate for changing attitudes and behaviour.

A general public information programme is nevertheless a necessary reinforcing agent for more specific education programmes. It is aimed at increasing an awareness of the size and complexity of the problem, which reinforces educational programmes, as well as reinforces political and legislative programmes[3]. It may start a chain reaction to strengthen the attack on many fronts. Public information also activates volunteers and contributors.

The media may be used to:

- Increase public awareness of the health consequences of smoking.

- Persuade adults to give up smoking, by rational argument.

- Influence youth generally.

- Create an atmosphere in which it is realised that smoking is not the normal or majority behaviour.

- Establish the rights of the non-smoker.

- Inform the public about the relative risks of pipes, cigars, low-tar cigarettes and less hazardous smoking habits.

- Inform government, politicians and the public about issues of basic policy.

- Publicise specific policy objectives in order to mobilise sympathetic public opinion and thereby to increase political pressure. (Timing is important here).

- Analyse and criticise aspects of tobacco industry activity.

- Counter inaccurate information and respond with accurate facts.

- Publicise success, obstacles and problems met by a programme.

- Provide information on availability of educational materials and smoking cessation activities.

- Discuss, emphasise and reinforce other programmes of interest.

Special care should be taken when deciding the message content. Fear-arousing or moralising approaches should be avoided. A non- or ex-smoker may feel happy in front of an intimidating poster, because this reinforces his intentions to refrain from smoking. But the current smoker's reality is different.

It is also worth while discussing the effect of pictures in the health education material. It is sometimes hard to distinguish an anti-smoker poster from a tobacco advertisement. Avoiding the same themes - smokers, ash-trays etc - may help in showing smoking as a minority behaviour, perhaps especially in countries where smoking is still fairly uncommon.

A public information campaign is obviously more reliable when its leaders are non-smokers. A cancer society should aim at smokeless environments starting with the society's own premises, meetings and press conferences.

A public information programme is a part of a more comprehensive community or nationwide smoking control programme. The latter is a part of a larger health-orientated programme in the community. The leaders of these various projects must therefore know about each other's activities to keep the message from over-lapping or conflicting. The boards and groups of a cancer society must also be informed in order to keep the various cancer messages from conflicting.

6.1.4.   Identifying Target Groups

As discussed in the preceding chapter it is important to tailor information and education according to the needs and situations of the various groups in the community. These groups differ from each other by age and sex, smoking history, social, ethnic and educational background etc. For an effective smoking-reduction programme these groups and their special needs must be identified. Not only does this help in designing the public information programme; it is also essential for planning and using specific health education methods; face-to-face education and education in groups.

General information about the health effects of smoking, the benefits and methods of cessation, the services to help people to stop smoking and legislative decisions may be directed to the public as a whole. However, an important step is to identify the persons and groups which can either support the programme or benefit from it. All these groups (government, health care personnel, media, schools, smokers, patients, parents, etc) also need a specific approach. Supported by public information and supplied with special information, training and skills, these people can be active in smoking reduction in their own surroundings - work and leisure. This includes among others legislation, persuasion of people to refrain from smoking, creating more services for those who need help in cessation, environmental change to create smoke-free surroundings, training in various components of the programme and exemplar action. The identification of specific target groups in the population is based on demographic data and data on smoking habits. To organise a demographic study is a relatively simple matter since[3]:

- Sampling methods are readily available and relatively familiar to any behavioural scientist (and every nation, developing or otherwise, has more than one such person).

- Protocols (questionnaires, interview schedules, rating scales, and so on) exist at present in many countries and with proper translation by a knowledgeable national translator would be ready for early use by the programmers with sensible alterations to fit the culture.

- Valuable data can quickly be accumulated by hand since protocol scoring is simple. Statistics can be worked on unsophisticated calculators; where computers exist, masses of sophisticated data can be processed in a short period of time.

- Interpretation of the basic data requires skills common in the repertoire of behavioural scientists.

- Research/data processing experts are available in many parts of the world and usually are anxious to help.

- A simple discussion of sampling techniques and a system of standardisation of measurement of smoking patterns has been prepared by a UICC Working Party[3].

The survey gives information on what groups need special smoking programmes. It may be found out for instance, that the smoking habit is especially widespread in children who have left school, in some occupational groups, in females of a limited age group, in urban surroundings etc. This knowledge helps to assess priorities and choose the content and methods of health information and education.

The same approach is useful when evaluating the programme. In all smoking control health education programmes it is advisable to use standardized measurements of smoking rates[3]. This enables international and national comparisons.

6.1.5.(i) Smoking Education - Young People

In the question of smoking, children are actually not free to choose. They are encouraged by their peers, adults, tobacco industry, films, TV-programmes and the overall climate of the society. Except for sales promotion this encouragement is not intentional, but may strongly influence the decision to start smoking. After an experimental phase smoking may become a habit.

Another point here is that smoking produces measurable health damage even at an early age.

Young people need truthful, interesting, positive and activating health education to refrain from smoking. This education should be integrated in the school curriculum. Special projects should be selected and planned with the help of the young people themselves. The range of fruitful approaches is wide indeed. But whatever is done, a great deal of effort should be aimed at diminishing the pressures towards smoking in society. It is very probable that the impact of a parent, pop star, teacher or athlete is greater than the net effect of an active smoking education programme limited to the child's school environment. "Do what I say" may have a minimal influence compared with the effect of a parent's smoking cessation.

Data-gathering on these matters and on the smoking habits of various groups of youngsters help to design the smoking-reducing approach. But educational efforts need support. Therefore it is evident that smoking in schools should not be allowed. Smoking by teachers should be limited to their offices. Tobacco products should not be sold to children under certain years of age. Non-smoking areas, buildings and vehicles should be arranged. Anti-smoking groups and other activities for youngsters could be arranged as well.

Young people should be helped to see non-smoking as an important part of their health behaviour. Education in schools could stress this, and teach decision-making skills. Information on the health hazards of smoking is needed, but the facts should form a clear entity and not just a basket of non-related loose facts. A positive and attractive image of a non-smoker should be built and the young people encouraged to resist peer-smoking influence. Practice in this denial may be as useful as the knowledge of the health hazards of smoking.

The situation of children at school differs from that of those youngsters who have already left school. The latter group generally smokes more. For instance, in Finland, 10 percent of 18-year olds in secondary school with a good performance smoked daily compared to 56 percent of those who had left school[12]. This reflects the great difference in these youngsters' situation and proves that smoking really is a many-faceted question. It also indicates the need for realism and careful choice of methods. Young people having left school and entered working life at an early age are hardly affected by the methods traditionally used in the schools. After identifying these groups and their sub-groups a face-to-face or a small group approach might be more fruitful. Often the only way to transmit the message to these youngsters is the media of which radio and television are the most popular among this age group.

6.1.5.(ii) Smoking Education - Adults

Smoking adults need support in their efforts to give up smoking. Non-smokers and especially ex-smokers need support in remaining non-smoking. A wide range of methods has been developed for adults. Parallel with the more general public information programmes, special target groups must be identified and special programmes designed. Such target groups could be:

- pregnant mothers, parents of young children

- exemplar groups (teachers, doctors, nurses etc)

- workers with occupational health hazards

- people with chronic illnesses

- clubs, societies

- etc

The needs and interests of these groups differ essentially from each other, and therefore special messages must be designed for each. The design may include delivering facts relevant to the situation of a special group, but may also include supportive means like withdrawal groups or therapies or face-to-face support from a skilled health educator.

The content of the message depends very much on the characteristics of the target group. Some general rules apply here. Fear-arousing messages must be carefully avoided especially where no possibilities for individual discussions exist. The reasons for smoking may be deeply rooted and difficult to oppose. Most smokers have long wanted to stop. The message should not therefore oversimplify or underestimate this problem or the difficulties people face when trying to stop smoking. Continuation of smoking is rarely a sign of too little information but rather a lack of relevant support. This support may be given by a professional. A group of people trying to stop smoking together often gives strong enough support. This helps in critical situations even outside the group meetings.

6.1.6. Changing the Climate of Opinion

Smoking has been considered a serious health problem in the developed countries for decades. Smoking threatens to become such a problem in the developing countries as well. In both cases public opinion can influence governments to do more to reduce the harmful effects of smoking. They could be influenced to implement legislation and to make tobacco prices keep pace with the general cost of living as well as to use price policy as a tool to make the industry develop less harmful products. Governments could be motivated to monitor the smoking habits of the population regularly and by this means evaluate the outcome of governmental and educational efforts. Smoke-free environments should be created and the rights of non-smokers respected.

When influencing the government facts on the effects of smoking, analysis of the costs due to smoking and a knowledge of international recommendations are valuable. A continuous public information programme may soften the attitudes of the opposing decision-makers, even the smoking ones. A public opinion survey - when favourable to government action against smoking - may strongly affect the government. Top medical and other experts can use their personal influence to persuade individual politicians and parties. Constructive propositions concerning the fate of tobacco cultivators and workers when smoking diminishes can be made. International positive experience on governmental action can be published.

An effective smoking control programme has many components supporting each other. Legislation to reduce the harmful effects of smoking is one of these. A Tobacco Act is not only a restrictive measure but may include protective components and acknowledge health education. Tobacco legislation could include:

- ensuring economic support to smoking reducing health education programmes
- limiting or prohibiting sales promotion
- controlling and regulating the tobacco products (maximum levels for tar etc) packages included
- health warnings in packages
- restrictions and prohibitions of smoking in certain places, vehicles etc
- restriction of tobacco sales (to young people)
- taxation and classification of the products on the basis of the yields of harmful components

In countries which have a comprehensive legislation the overall experience is encouraging. More time is needed to assess the long-term impact of these laws. By legislation governments confirm to the public that the smoking questions are to be taken seriously. Legislation also enables a more comprehensive smoking control.

The degree of health hazards and nicotine dependence is a function of the inhaled doses of the harmful components in the smoke. By low tar programmes the risk can be reduced in theory. However, a low tar programme must not undermine efforts to stop smoking altogether. It is possible to manufacture cigarettes low in tar and nicotine. In low tar cigarettes the amounts of several substances like acrolein, cyanide and formaldehyde are low as well. Carbon monixide can be low or high in the so called low tar products. It seems that a light cigarette should give a low tar and carbon monoxide yield, but is still not low in nicotine. The tobacco industry can control these things, but control is less feasible in the case of products other than cigarettes. In countries where low tar products are available and familiar their share is increasing.

Changing from high tar to low tar products, leaving a long butt, avoiding inhaling the smoke and smoking fewer cigarettes a day help to diminish the risks of smoking. A low tar programme is only part of the smoking control programme; but its main role is to encourage people to give up smoking.

A low tar programme starts by controlling and regulating tar, nicotine and carbon monoxide levels in the market and possibly abolishing the very high tar brands. The results of these measurements must be published. Cigarettes can be classified according to the yields of their harmful components and this classification may be used as a basis for taxation and public information. The public can be encouraged to choose a less hazardous cigarette and not to smoke more or inhale more after changing the brand. The utmost objective is always to reduce the diseases due to smoking and this must be constantly emphasized in the low tar programme.

Rights of Non-Smokers

Smoking is usually a minority behaviour. Symptoms caused by involuntary (passive) smoking and the recent mounting evidence on the possibility of passive smoking-related lung cancer have strengthened the movement against smoking. It is no longer right to consider smoking to be one's own business only. Apart from health effects, smoking causes involuntary economic losses to the tax payers.

It can therefore be predicted that the non-smoking majority will in the future act more in a majority fashion. Several associations for non-smokers' rights have been founded. These are active in influencing governments, other decision-makers and the public. The rights of non-smokers are much discussed in those working places where involuntary smoking is common. Conflicts in these matters are common, too. There are also countries with associations for the smokers' rights.

In the long run smoking will turn out to be a transitory phenomenon in the world. It may disappear totally during the next century. In the meantime strong and effective smoking-reducing

programmes are needed. Stressing and respecting non-smokers' rights
is one part of the control programme. A smoke-free society is an
important goal but not at the expense of the mental health of
society and its members' ability to co-operate with each other in
other health issues. Serious social conflicts in smoking matters
should not be aroused, or at least their widespread effects
carefully considered beforehand.

6.1.7.   *Smoking Cessation Programmes*

For every smoker stopping is worthwhile. We know that the
excess risk of lung cancer is lost after ten years of non-smoking[7].
In bladder cancer at least seven years of non-smoking is required
to minimise the excess risk[13]. The bronchial epithelium recovers
structurally in people who stop smoking for over two years[14]. The
risk of cardiovascular diseases diminishes considerably in a few
years as well[2].

There is now a large body of knowledge on the economic and
social benefits of quitting smoking. Most smokers want to stop.
The smoker's own desire and motivation is of course a prerequisite
and not much is gained by trying to push those who are not yet
prepared to stop.

The decision to stop smoking can be helped and supported in
many ways. The key-persons here are health-care workers, family
members and friends including cancer society volunteers. Most
smokers who stop do so without any help from an organized
cessation activity, probably encouraged by others. The considerable
effect of mutual encouragement can be exploited by encouraging the
formation of self-help groups of smokers who want to quit.

Smoking cessation programmes among adults and youth have
produced somewhat contradictory results. Education programmes
for adults have included various smoking cessation clinics and a
variety of more specific withdrawal methods. These methods have
included individual counselling, emotional role playing, aversive
conditioning, desensitization and specific techniques to reduce
the likelihood that smoking will occur in situations previously
associated with smoking. Some of these techniques have produced
poor results, while studies of other methods have shown inconsistent
results. The two methods showing the most promise are individual
counselling and smoking withdrawal clinics[15].

A highly effective resource in smoking control may not yet
be used often enough. This is the simple and persuasive advice
given by doctors to their smoking patients. A large proportion
of the population visits general practitioners at least once
in five years. In one study a group of patients was advised to
stop smoking. They were given a leaflet to help them and they
were also told that they would be followed up. Over 5 percent of
this group of patients stopped smoking during the first month and
were still not smoking one year after[16]. If every general
practitioner were to adopt this practice the actual numbers of
smokers quitting the habit would be very large indeed.

Smoking withdrawal clinics and groups give long term support to those who want to stop smoking. Withdrawal symptoms, benefits of stopping, weight gain, relaxation, and other crucial topics can be tackled in the clinics and groups. Hypnosis, acupuncture and psychotherapy have been used to support people in their efforts to be and remain an ex-smoker. The overall results vary from 20 percent to 60 percent. Whatever the frame and method is, it is important to serve the needs of the target group. Experts are needed in planning and implementing these programmes. One role of a Cancer Society is to experiment with these methods and try to find solutions for an adequate support for those who want to stop smoking.

REFERENCES

1.   Atkinson, A.B. and Townsend, J.L. : Economic Aspects of
        Reduced Smoking. Lancet, Vol 2, 8036 : 492-494, 1977.

2.   Report of a WHO Expert Committee : Smoking and its effects
        on Health. World Health Organization, Technical Report
        Series 568, Geneva 1975.

3.   Gray, N. and Daube, M. : Guidelines for Smoking Control.
        2nd Edition UICC Technical Report Series, 52, Geneva 1980.

4.   Redmond Jr, D.E. : Tobacco and Cancer, The First Clinical
        Report 1761. New Engl. J. Med. 282 : 18-23, 1970.

5.   Hirayama, T. : Non-smoking Wives of Heavy Smokers Have a
        Higher Risk of Lung Cancer. A Study from Japan. Brit.
        Med. Jnl. Vol 282, 183-185, 1981.

6.   Trichopoulos, D., Kalandidi, A., Sparros, L. and MacMahon, B.
        Lung Cancer and Passive Smoking. Int. J. Cancer 27, 1-4,
        1981.

7.   Doll, R. and Peto, R. : Mortality in Relation to Smoking :
        20 Years Observations on Male British Doctors. Brit. Med.
        Jnl. 4, 1525-1536, 1976.

8.   Laszlo, G., Archer, G.G., Darrell, J.H., Dawson, J.M. and
        Fletcher, C.M. : The Diagnosis and Prophylaxis of
        Pulmonary Complications of Surgical Operation. Brit. J.
        Surg. 60, 129-134, 1973.

9.   Shaw, H.M. and Milton, G.W. : Smoking and the Development
        of Metastases from Malignant Melanoma. Int. J. Cancer 28,
        153-156, 1981.

10.   Daniell, H.W. : Breast Cancer and Smoking. World Smoking
        and Health 5, 46, 1980.

11.   Johnston-Early, A. et al. : Smoking Abstinence and Small
        Cell Lung Cancer Survival. An Association. JAMA 244,
        2175-2179, 1980.

12.   Rimpelä, M. : Tupakoinnin alkaminen. Incidence of Smoking
        among Finnish Youth - a Follow-up Study, Tampere 1980.

13.   Skrabanek, P. and Walsh, A. : Bladder Cancer, UICC Technical
Report Series, Vol 60, Geneva 1981.

14.   Bertram, J.F. and Rogers, A.W. : Recovery of Bronchial
Epithelium on Stopping Smoking. Brit. Med. Jnl. 283,
1567-1569, 1981.

15.   Thompson, E.L. : Smoking Education Programmes 1960 - 1976.
Am. Jnl. Pub. Hlth. 68, 250-257, 1978.

16.   Russell, M.A.H., Wilson, C., Taylor, C. and Baker, C.D. :
Effects of General Practitioners' Advice Against Smoking.
Brit. Med. Jnl. 2, 231-235, 1979.

CHAPTER 7 - PUBLIC RELATIONS

INTRODUCTION

Public relations has been defined as "the state of mutual understanding between an organization or individual and any groups of persons or organizations and the extent of quality of the reputation that exists". This definition is clear, but for the purposes of this guide it can be translated as a working philosophy into "the deliberate, planned and sustained effort to establish and maintain mutual understanding between a national cancer society and its public". Every successful cancer society will wish to take whatever actions are necessary to ensure that good and mutually beneficial relationships with others are well maintained. The actions which it takes to secure publicity must be deliberate and shaped in such a way to draw attention to certain facts and stimulate a desire to assist financially. In the following pages the general principles of public relations and the methods used in gaining publicity are dealt with in detail; however, no guide can possibly cover every situation which may arise and those involved in the cancer society must be constantly aware of the need for continuing publicity and always be ready to seize every opportunity that may arise.

7.1. GENERAL PRINCIPLES OF PUBLIC RELATIONS

7.1.1. Public Recognition of the Cancer Society

Many cancer societies undervalue the importance of good publicity and public relations. It is imagined that organizing publicity is a complicated business which will require time and effort which would be better spent getting on with the job in hand. It is argued that good works and achievements will speak for themselves and that the organization is well known anyway. Sadly, this is a common error. Most people have busy lives to lead and only a tiny proportion of them will get involved in the activities of the local cancer society. Certainly they will often give, and give generously when approached, but in most countries there are a very large number of such organizations all competing with each other for the public's attention and generosity. It will be necessary, therefore, to ensure that the cancer society maintains its position in the public eye and continues to attract its share of their support.

7.1.2. Publicity

The most basic reason for publicity is to communicate information about an organization or a cause to the widest possible effect. However, within this general aim several objectives can be identified.

- To attract additional resources such as money, new members or volunteers.

- To attract people to particular events such as public meetings or fundraising functions.

- To campaign on, or inform people about certain issues.

-   To strengthen the morale of the organization.

Of course publicity does not necessarily need such specific aims as those outlined above. Many of the day-to-day activities of a cancer society will probably be of general interest to the public at large. Indeed, people often complain that newspapers, radio and television programmes give far too much coverage to bad news and not enough to the positive things happening in the community, or to issues of social and community concern. While there may be some truth in this point of view, the fault often lies as much with the cancer society and other voluntary organizations, as it does with the media. It is not enough to expect the media to come and search out matters of community concern. They must be made aware of what organizations are doing. Thus publicity is something which the cancer society must seek, to ensure that the community is kept informed of its existence, activities and need for continuing support.

Another important reason for cancer societies to concentrate more on publicity is to break down the isolation that many of their volunteers and support groups working in different parts of the country may feel. Often these volunteers and local committees or groups are working in relative isolation and the publicity about the success of the societies' work is likely to encourage and stimulate their efforts.

Thus publicity must have three elements to be successful: There must be:

-   short term publicity to highlight immediate achievements,
-   continuing publicity about current projects, campaigns and programmes,
-   long term publicity about long term goals, i.e. the prospects of finding cures for cancers, of achieving higher success rates from early treatment or the goal of building a new research institute.

Any good public relations programme should, therefore, be planned to include elements of short term, continuing and long term goals for the organization.

It is not possible to mention here all the events and activities which justify special public relations or publicity activity by the cancer society. However, important opportunities to attract attention to the society and its objectives are sometimes overlooked. Press releases on scientific advances help at fundraising campaign time. Announcements of new developments in treatment attract attention and create an awareness of the cancer problem. Stories of cured cancer patients and the importance of early detection also make good copy. Services to cancer patients and exciting research advances are also good for stories. Educational forums, film showings and exhibitions all stir interest in the media. There are opportunities to make prestige awards to distinguished scientists or clinicians and the opportunity to give recognition for long service to the society by volunteers and committee members. Publicity about long service or prestige awards helps to highlight the work that is constantly going on in the background for the society and also to stimulate and motivate other volunteers. They are, moreover, human interest stories which the press and media are always more willing to give their attention to.

7.1.3. *Target Audiences for Public Relations*

The cancer society, to be truly effective in its public relations and publicity activities, must plan the target audiences which it intends its message to reach. These will generally be:

- the subscriber and volunteer
- the general public
- patients
- scientists and health professionals

A planned public relations programme, once the objectives and the publicity theme have been agreed, is more than a list of actions to be taken. It almost always requires these actions to be organized so that they may be controlled, timed and evaluated as projects. A public relations programme will usually include several of such projects.

If publicity to subscribers is felt to be one method of achieving the desired objectives, a project might be to ensure a steady flow of information to these subscribers every month of the year. If, on the other hand, the need was to establish a new corporate identity for the cancer society following re-organization or a change in policies then a long term project could perhaps be a total re-design of every facet of the society's visual presentation, i.e. literature, visual aids, posters, etc. A short term project could be a news conference to ensure that journalists and media personnel understood the cancer society's structure and aims and objectives. Within the total timetable of the public relations programme, each project would have its own timetable. This permits an accurate assessment to be made of the progress of the campaign which should be carefully monitored by those responsible within the cancer society. Bearing in mind the four target audiences already specified, it might be that the cancer society would decide that subscribers and volunteers should be kept informed and motivated by regular information on progress on fund-raising and in the achievement of campaign objectives. The general public on the other hand would be more likely to be interested in the overall situation concerning cancer, the potential for prevention and early diagnosis and treatment, and any major advances that may occur in the field of cancer.

Patients are likely to be interested in information concerning rehabilitation programmes and facilities for treatment which are provided by the cancer society. Scientists and clinicians are likely to be interested in any contribution the cancer society may make to the provision of research or treatment facilities and in professional symposia organized, as well as receiving copies of specialist publications from the cancer society.

It is worth emphasizing the importance of ensuring that target audiences and objectives for one's public relations and publicity strategy are clearly defined.

7.1.4.   *Budgeting the Public Relations Programme*

The cancer society must decide just how much money can be spent on the public relations programme because this will largely determine the methods that can be used. On a limited budget it will not be possible to produce glossy publications in which to sell the society and usually it will exclude the use of paid newspaper and media advertising. However, it is wrong to make the mistake that an effective public relations programme must cost large amounts of money. Nevertheless, it is important for the cancer society to realise that it will be necessary to make adequate provision in their overall budget for public relations. Some of the items which must be included in this budget will be:

- The cost of a public relations officer or public relations consultancy and the cost of travelling and expenses incurred by them.

- Press conferences, including the cost of accommodation, refreshments and hospitality.

- Press releases and the cost of special stationery and postage' and maintenance of a proper press list.

- The cost of photographs and photographic services.

- Media monitoring, i.e. the cost of press cutting services, radio and television transcripts and subscriptions to papers and periodicals.

- Special public relations events when campaigns are launched.

- Temporary services - it is sometimes necessary to call on temporary executive or secretarial help to carry out particular public relations or publicity jobs.

- Films and exhibitions - such must be carefully accounted and included in the budget.

- Direct mail - an important part of any cancer society's public relations programme, the cost of postage, etc, must be allowed, as well as that of the secretarial work involved in putting direct mail letters together.

- Telephone calls, telex, telegrams, etc, must also be accounted for in the budget.

It is important to realise that once a budget has been established, it will dictate the broad scope of work for the coming year. It will be necessary and important to keep a check on expenditure. Naturally a budget cannot cover every eventuality and it is for this reason that it should contain a sufficient reserve for unforseen contingencies. However, this should not be an excuse for sloppy, uncontrolled forecasting. A periodic review of the cost effectiveness of the organization's public relations campaign should be carried out. It is important for any voluntary

organization to have value for money and to be sure that
expenditure on specific promotional activities is justified by the
return, bearing in mind that although publicity efforts alone do
not raise money, they do inspire and motivate the public to support
the cancer society.

7.2.   ORGANIZATION OF A PUBLIC RELATIONS PROGRAMME

7.2.1.   Public Relations Committee

Public relations and publicity is such an important component
of the cancer society's activities that it should be a special
responsibility of one of the committees of the organization. It
may well be that this responsibility will be included in the remit
of an education and information committee or it may be that a
separate publicity committee would be formed. In either case it
is helpful to enlist the support of journalists from newspaper and
broadcasting media to serve on these committees. It is also of
vital importance that the chief executive of the cancer society
ensures close liaison between all those concerned with projecting
the organization's public relations image and disseminating
information about cancer. To be avoided at all costs is any
confusion in the various messages projected in the publicity, fundraising or public education activities of the cancer society.
Emotive statements about cancer and its curability may make the
headlines but may be detrimental to the overall educational
objectives.

7.2.2.   Public Relations Officer

Every cancer society should have one full-time member of
staff responsible for public relations and publicity. This may in
some small organization be combined with other duties, however the
individual holding this appointment must be a skilled communicator
able to establish good relationships with the press and media and
ideally with journalistic skills. He or she should work under the
direction of the chief executive and have close liaison with all
those responsible for the activities of the cancer society so that
they are able to advise on opportunities which arise for publicity.
It should be the role of the public relations and publicity
officer to seize every opportunity to gain space and time in the
media at no cost or at least a very marginal cost to the cancer
society. Indeed, an essential quality of this individual will be
that of opportunist since many day-to-day opportunities for
publicity will arise without prior notice and must be seized.

7.2.3.   Public Relations Agency

In many countries professional public relations agencies or
consultants are available on a fee basis to the cancer society.
The growth of awareness of public relations and the increase in
the number of practitioners has been phenomenal over the past
twenty five years. There are both advantages and disadvantages in
using a public relations consultancy. The breadth of experience
of the professional consultant enables them to evaluate and apply
usually sound judgment to a wide range of communications,
opportunities and problems. The consultancy's resources in terms

of people also gives it flexibility in carrying out the work. Some
organizations use consultancies to obtain an independent outside view
and a wider range of experience, skill and talent than would normally
be available economically within a single organization. Many of
the professional public relations consultancies subscribe to a
code of practice such as those belonging to an Institute of Public
Relations. However, it may often be that the cancer society's
budget will not permit the hiring of the services of professional
consultants whose fees are likely to be substantial. In this, as
in all things, the organization must decide where it will get the
most value for money commensurate with keeping expenditure on
publicity and fundraising to acceptable limits.

7.2.4.   *Public Relations Concerns All*

In the discussion about public relations officers, consultants,
agencies and committees, it has been the intention to demonstrate
that good public relations and effective publicity do not happen
by chance and must be approached in an organized fashion. However,
it is important to realise that every individual and group working
with, and for the cancer society will affect the image of the
organization and thus must accept responsibility for public relations
in their words and deeds. For example, one volunteer acting in
an irresponsible manner can generate a great deal of bad publicity
for the cancer society. Conversely, if every staff member and
volunteer is aware of the potential for good public relations then
they can do much to maximise on every opportunity to promote the
cancer society and its work.

7.3.   *PLANNING PUBLIC RELATIONS ACTIVITIES*

7.3.1.   *Organizing a Press Conference*

The organization of a press or news conference is standard
practice when a story needs amplification or explanation to a
group of journalists. Before calling a conference ensure that it
is worthwhile and necessary. If all the facts can be explained
in a press release, even if it needs some pages of background
material attached to it, there is no need to call a conference.
If the cancer society does not wish to give any further information
or explanation than that which is already included in their
written release, it is pointless to ask journalists to spend
valuable time on what may turn out to be a non-event.

Technically there is a difference between a news conference,
a press briefing and a press reception. Normally a news conference
is called when there is some important specific item of news to
announce. A briefing may be held to ensure that journalists and
others understand the background to some event or development. A
press reception, on the other hand, is normally held when the news
to be announced is what is described as "soft" - some internal
development within the cancer society, the launch of a new service
or even the appointment of a new council or staff member. Most
press conferences can be planned well ahead and it is normal
practice for ten or fourteen days' notice of events to be given.
This will enable journalists to put the event into their diary
for that week and also give editors time to decide whether to send
a reporter to cover the event or not.

Just before the press conference a check should be made to
see if a representative is being sent by the newspaper or media
concerned and even if not, arrangements can be made to send the
news editor concerned a press release about the occasion. Advance
notice is usually given in the form of a press invitation or in the
form of a letter giving brief but complete details of what the
event is about. A useful rule of thumb is the 'what, why, who and
where' approach. What is to be said, i.e. the message. Why it is
being said, i.e. the purpose. Who it is desired to reach, i.e.
the intended audience. And where they can be reached, i.e. the
outlets.

Carefully select the timing and location for the event, both
day of week and time of day. In doing so it should be borne in
mind the needs of daily, weekly and monthly papers and similarly
the requirements of radio and television commentators. It is also
important, if possible, to try to avoid clashing with any other
press conferences which may be planned for that day.

Ensure that the location is suitable and that there are
adequate facilities in the room chosen to hold the conference or
reception. It is good procedure to get all those attending to
sign a visitors' book so that newspapers and media not represented
may afterwards be sent a copy of the press release issued. It is
useful when facilities permit for the cancer society concerned to
hold the press receptions and conferences at their headquarters to
give identity to the cancer society. If this is not possible
because of limitations of space, the facilities of the local
hospital or cancer treatment centre may sometimes be utilized to
advantage.

7.3.2.   Preparing Press Releases

To ensure accurate and regular coverage of the activities of
the cancer society by the media it is essential to produce good
press releases which are interesting, concise and properly laid
out. Two things go towards making a good press release - content
and technique.

Content

Any news item must revolve around five major facts, i.e.
what happened, when, where and to whom. All press releases
should contain such information and preferably in the first
paragraph. The release should be as interesting and news-
worthy as possible. News about people, especially if they
are well known, is of interest. Human interest, suspense,
controversy, progress and the unusual are all subjects
likely to be interesting. Imagination must be used in
making a release as topical and as interesting as possible.
However, stick to the facts and keep the release as simple
as possible. The media can always come back to the cancer
society if they want further details. Also make sure that
facts and opinions are carefully segregated.

Technique

It should always be remembered that the aim is to make
the job of the reporter or sub-editor as easy as possible.

The less a story is cut or re-written, the less
likelihood there is of its meaning being changed.
Also it is most likely that something which requires
no work will be printed.

- The Basic Sheet - Keep the release to one sheet of paper
whenever possible. If a second page is absolutely necessary,
use a second sheet, not the back of the first sheet. Paper
size - use a standard paper, preferably A4. It is also
useful to have the cancer society's name, address and logo
on the press release paper so that it will be instantly
recognisable as being a news release from your organization.

- Headline - Give the release a title which indicates its content
and purpose. It must be typed in capitals and there should be
reasonable space between the title and the opening line of the
release.

- First Paragraph - The first paragraph of a release is of the
utmost importance and should emphasize the message indicated
in the headline.

- Identification - It is essential to make sure that the name
and address and telephone number of an individual to whom
enquiries may be addressed is given at the end of the release.

- Underlining - Never underline anything in a press release - not
even on the headline. This indicates to the printer that the
words underlined are to be printed in italic.

- Capitals - Use only capital letters for titles or proper names.

- Typing - Releases should always be typed with double spacing
with additional space between paragraphs. There should be
margins of at least 1½" (4 cm) on either side.

- Paragraphs - All new paragraphs should be indented two spaces.
Paragraphs should be kept short and easily read.

- Date - Always give the date of issue on a release.

- Embargo - This is an instruction to the press that the story
is not to be published before a certain date and sometimes even
a certain time on that date. An embargo should be avoided if
possible. If an embargo is requested make the reason clear.
It should appear above the title on the first page.

- Photographs - If photographs are available this can be stated
on the release. Details should come after the body of the
story and the author's name. Every picture should have a
piece of paper attached giving captions and other details.
Action photographs of people doing things are much more
effective than posed scenes.

7.3.3.   *Interviews with Journalists*

The cancer society should always be prepared, and indeed
actively encourage interviews with journalists to give them indepth

knowledge about topics of interest concerning cancer. Obviously
it is valuable to cultivate a good relationship with local
journalists and media commentators and one way of doing this is
to provide an information service for them. Always be prepared
to give them help and advice when they are compiling a story on
a topic which concerns the cancer society. However, caution is
always necessary when discussing any matter with journalists since
anything that the representative of the cancer society says is
likely to be quoted.

If cancer societies maintain an information, resource centre
and library then they should make this facility known to local
journalists and media personnel since this can be a valuable
resource to them when they are researching articles and features.

7.3.4. *Broadcasts on Radio and Television*

A result of good relationships with the local media can
often result in the cancer society being asked to comment on
topical news items on radio and television. It may also involve
cancer society personnel in other broadcasts such as documentary
programmes on cancer-related topics, on radio phone-ins and in
broadcasts about the organization's current activities which may
have been stimulated by press conferences or press releases issued
by the society. There is neither the space nor time here to
discuss broadcasting techniques, however, it is well worthwhile
for cancer societies to train key staff members and other spokesmen
in the art of radio and television speaking. Personnel who may be
good communicators in front of an audience or in a lecture
situation can sometimes "dry up" when put in a live broadcast
situation or be subject to aggressive questioning by a media
interviewer. Remember, the potential for publicity which exists
in media interviews is worth large amounts of paid advertising,
usually way beyond the means of the local cancer society. It pays
to seek out every possible opportunity for such free media time.

7.3.5. *Public talks*

Most cancer societies will frequently be invited to speak
at public meetings ; either those which they arrange themselves
or at meetings of other voluntary organizations and societies.
It is important to have a format for such talks which presents in
a concise form the aims, objectives and services operated by the
cancer society. The aim will be not just to inform people, but
to either educate them about cancer and thus create a change in
their attitude to the disease, or to enlist their support for
your activities. It should be remembered that the status of the
speaker will affect their credibility, so ensure that those who
give public talks on behalf of the cancer society have the
authority and standing to impress the audience. Face-to-face
communications in such a situation is one of the most valuable
methods of promoting the cancer society's work since it permits
questions and answers from the audience, an element missing in
printed communication and most broadcast communications media.
The contact made with the public at such talks is also invaluable
in the opportunity it presents to place in their hands the
literature which the cancer society has produced.

7.3.6. Recorded Messages

Several countries have found that recorded telephone messages can be used to good effect in promoting the work of the cancer society and making known the facilities that it offers to the community. If the telephone facilities permit, then cancer societies will find that there is value in utilizing recorded messages.

7.3.7. Displays and Exhibitions

Valuable opportunities exist to promote the cancer society's work through exhibitions and displays. These might be either displays organized in connection with public meetings which the cancer society is holding, or larger events such as Ideal Home Exhibitions and similar events which are now featured at large exhibition and conference centres in many countries. At a lower key, displays can be usefully organized in shop windows, libraries or even on streets on busy shopping days.

Sometimes the cancer society is fortunate enough to have a mobile display unit which can be of tremendous value in promoting the work of the organization and taking it to the public in areas which would otherwise not be accessible to their message. As with other forms of publicity, the cancer society should be clear on just what its aim is with any such exhibition or display. It might be to publicise the cancer society, to recruit volunteers or to focus attention on the treatment, early detection or diagnosis of cancer. The material should be chosen carefully accordingly. It takes time to organize a good exhibition and it may also require professional advice and facilities if these are not available within the cancer society. Remember that the image projected by such a display or exhibition will again affect the corporate image of the organization as a whole.

7.3.8. Audio-Visual Aids

The value of exhibitions and displays can often be enhanced by good audio-visual material. Most cancer societies will use films or slides in the course of their public education work. It may not always be possible to have a film made about the cancer society since this will cost a considerable sum of money. However, most cancer societies will be able to use slides depicting their work and this can often be incorporated into a display panel for use at exhibitions. Such slide presentations are also of great value in promoting the society's image when public talks are given. Recorded messages have already been discussed and the more sophisticated tape/slide presentations which are available these days are usually within the financial reach of most cancer societies; in the absence of colour/sound films, these can provide a sophisticated media for the projection of the cancer society's message.

Increasing interest in recent years has been given to closed circuit television as an economic method of conveying messages to the public. Facilities exist in many educational establishments, schools, hospitals and commercially for closed circuit television and the cancer society should explore the possibilities of using such facilities to produce material for its own use.

7.3.9.   *Literature and Posters*

The range of literature and posters which individual cancer societies may produce will depend on the scope of their activities, but since many cancer societies will be involved in education and care, they are likely to produce a number of different leaflets and posters. The quality of the material produced is important in that it will once again reflect on the cancer society. Remember, in many cases such literature may be the only opportunity the cancer society has of presenting its image and message to certain sections of the community. Their response is likely to be affected by the impression that they receive from such literature. Clearly, as cancer societies are in large part funded from voluntary sources their literature should not appear to be excessively expensive to produce. The glossy publications of large commercial organizations would be quite inappropriate; however, having said that, it is equally invidious to promote the opposite image of a cheap, poorly produced piece of literature which will reflect inefficiency and amateurism to readers.

Obviously as important as the general appearance is the content of such literature. Factually it must always be accurate, avoid over emotionalism in its tone and not seek to arouse fear in order to generate support from the public. The same rules apply to posters. Various publications produced by the cancer society will probably range in scope from simple advisory leaflets about various cancer topics to scientific publications. All of these will be valuable in projecting the image of the cancer society in different spheres. It is helpful, however, to have a "house style" for all publications produced. These will help to promote the society's corporate image and give an identity to all its printed material.

7.3.10.   *Annual Report*

The annual report of the cancer society is probably the most important piece of literature it is likely to produce. It will be read by scientists, clinicians, volunteers and supporters throughout the community. It will record the cancer society's progress and also probably contain many other informative articles. A very important section of this annual report will be the financial statement with records of funds raised over the previous twelve months. It is important to see that this annual report is circulated widely to all those who have contributed to the cancer society. Not only does it let them see that proper accountability is being made by the cancer society of funds raised, but will also help to stimulate further giving.

The annual report is also a useful document to acquaint potential new supporters with the scope and range of activities and services offered by the cancer society. Once again the same rules apply - over-glossy expensive publications will tend to suggest to potential supporters that the cancer society is spending unnecessary funds on printing. However, an image of professionalism must be projected so a good standard of presentation is required.

7.3.11.   Newsletter

Most cancer societies find that a newsletter which is circulated among volunteers and supporters and other interested personnel is of great value in keeping motivation high and informing people about their activities. Again this can help to stimulate publicity and a good news-sheet can be a very effective way of making the cancer society better known and publicising its activities. Preparing a newsletter can be a time-consuming occupation and sometimes after the first few issues it can be difficult to find material. Thus it is often better to produce an occasional newsletter when there is enough material rather than trying to produce it to a deadline on a very regular basis. It is important that such newsletters should be entertaining and read-able as well as informative. It is useful to invite contributions from people outside your organization who are nevertheless working on cancer related programmes.

7.3.12.   Advisory Literature

Education advisory literature will be dealt with elsewhere in this manual. However, it is important to mention in this section on public relations that literature used in one's education programme also effects the so-called corporate image of the cancer society and attention must be paid to this as well as the educational facts presented.

7.3.13.   Advertising

Cancer societies sometimes require paid advertising for their organization. The cost effectiveness of such advertising must be established beforehand and strict adherence to a prepared budget is necessary. It may be that the cancer society wishes to promote its education programme or some of its other services and feels that the use of selected journals, newspapers or even radio and television advertising is justified. On other occasions it may be desired to announce public meetings, recruit new volunteers or encourage subscriptions during a fundraising campaign. Once again it is vitally important to budget carefully since such advertising is very expensive. Sometimes local newspapers, which will cost much less than the large national newspapers, are more effective for the cancer society.

Careful research is required before planning any such advertising campaign and the advice of a professional advertising agency might well be necessary. The possibilities for advertising to a cancer society are widespread. Not only can press and broadcast media be used, but outside poster hoardings, posters or audio-visual displays, in railway stations, airports, new shopping precincts and hypermarkets are also possible, as are moving displays on the sides of buses or on undergrounds and trains. The scope today for advertising is enormous and the public relations/publicity officer of the cancer society must choose the most effective media to promote the society's special needs.

One other vitally important method of promoting the cancer
society's work is the direct mail letter. This method is valuable,
particularly in fundraising, but is subject to certain dangers.
Too often the response that such an approach might elicit would be
"Oh dear, another circular" and into the wastepaper basket it goes.
How can the cancer society ensure that people will read the letters
it sends out? Many books have been written about direct mail and
the art of writing the right letter to the right people, whether
it is to ten or to ten thousand. All kinds of special printing
techniques have been evolved for the purpose, especially in the
world of selling. It is useful to know something of modern printing
techniques and to perhaps seek advice from experts but the cancer
society can achieve a lot through using normal judgment, commonsense
and logic.

Direct mail letters should be of interest to the individual
personally and their curiosity must be aroused before they will
exert themselves to read it. Certainly if a letter is to persuade
people to send some of their hard earned money to the cancer society
they may know little about, it has to be exceptionally skillful in
its composition. Here are some of the main points which should be
borne in mind when composing such a letter:

- Simplicity - the language must be such that it can be understood
  by anyone and yet be dignified. It should be on one page. Both
  sentences and paragraphs should be kept short.

- A note of urgency or crisis should, where possible, be introduced
  when one is appealing for funds.

- Specific - the reader should be asked to take some specific
  action and reference should be made to an enclosure since
  the cancer society will wish to enclose a leaflet about its
  work with such a direct mail letter.

- Personal Touch - every letter, if it is to be effective, has
  to be shaped so that it is personal to the recipient. To be
  of real value the letter must be "topped and tailed", i.e.
  addressed Dear Mr Jones and signed personally by the writer.
  Duplicated signatures and forms of address such as 'Dear Sir
  or Madam' are to be avoided at all costs.

Clearly the value of the letter will be greatly enhanced if
it is signed by some well known and respected figure in the
community. It should be remembered that even with a good direct
mail shot, the response rate may only be as high as five per cent.
Nevertheless, this can still be very cost effective if the address
list is carefully selected.

7.4.   *CONCLUSION*

It has been said that the public are divided into three sets
of individuals. Those who are aware of what the cancer society
is attempting to do, and support it. Those who are aware of the
cancer society but do not support it, and those who neither know
of the society, nor support it. Unfortunately this latter group
is likely to be the majority and perhaps the most important aim

in public relations for a cancer society is to reach a position where those who support the society continue to do so, those who know about the society and do not at present support it, should start to give their support and that group who have never heard of the society and, therefore, cannot help it, should learn about its objectives and join the other two groups in giving support. When this happens the society will have achieved its public relations goals. However, even in the unlikely event that this ideal state of affairs was ever reached, then the cancer society would have to continue to work as hard as ever at maintaining the position. Public relations must always be a day-to-day concern of the successful cancer society, its committees, staff and volunteers, and equal in importance to every other activity in which they may engage.

CHAPTER 8 - FUNDRAISING

INTRODUCTION

People's health, because it is a personal concern, must be more than a government policy, more than just a government activity. It is to a large extent a people's business in which citizens must learn to protect their own health and to involve themselves with the health of their fellow men. Thus volunteer participation in health programmes through voluntary organizations is not merely desirable but essential.

Demands on governments often make it impossible for them adequately to finance health programmes. Funds from voluntary organizations not only supplement such programmes but pound for pound are more effective because they are backed by personal commitment. Such health programmes can also be much more flexible simply because they are independent. They can add valuable services to government and other health programmes with monies raised by and with the participation of volunteers. People have been raising funds for voluntary organizations for thousands of years. Indeed, the practice of charity is as old as mankind and has become instinctive. Modern inventions have transformed our way of life. Indeed, with the complexity of speed and the sometimes artificial character of modern life in the western world commuting between work and suburbia, hardship and distress tend to be hidden. At the same time, with the vast increases there have been in population of most countries, social problems are generally too large to be tackled by just one or two people on their own. So that to keep up with the revolution in living and to help with both old and new problems voluntary effort like everything else has had to be organized.

In the last century it was usual for charity to be the good works of a few wealthy individuals. However, the distribution of wealth within countries is changing and taxation often inhibits substantial giving by the wealthier individual. Today commerce and industry are assuming an increasing importance to charities as is a growing population with a higher standard of living and money to spare. As a first principle in fundraising therefore, it can be assumed that in most countries there exists a society which is prepared to be charitable. This section of the guide deals with ways in which the cancer society can best tap that reservoir of generosity.

There are certain principles, however, which have first to be established. First of all if a cancer society is appealing to the public for funds to support its programme it must ensure that the methods which it uses do not contain emotive or inaccurate messages in order to solicit the public's help. As discussed in Chapters 5 and 7, it is vitally important for a unified message to reach the public from the cancer society, a message which is harmonised between the education and information services, the fundraisers and those who are seeking publicity for the overall work of the society. If members of the public believe they have discovered untruths in statements made by the cancer society, they might justifiably suspect everything that is said with serious

81

effects on the overall aims of the society. Remember that fear is often the cause of delay in obtaining treatment for cancer so that adding to fears is likely to exacerbate this problem. Over-optimism also is not justifiable. Inaccurate statements such as "with early treatment all cancer is curable" is likely in the long term to result in disillusionment. Accuracy is essential.

It is worth mentioning also that, in fundraising, the example set by volunteers working with the cancer society can have a very powerful motivating effect on others in the community. It should, therefore, be a first principle that all volunteers support the work of the society financially. What people do, after all, speaks louder than what they say and the example set by a fundraising campaign chairman and his or her committee members who will usually be influential members of the community, can serve to stimulate their friends and business associates into equally generous giving.

Finally, and most importantly, it should be remembered that before launching any public appeal for funds the cancer society should arrange to discuss their objectives with the government. Indeed, government may itself be prepared to make substantial grants towards the achievement of their objectives. It is far better also that the cancer society be seen to be working in harmony or, better still, partnership with the government in its efforts to deal with the cancer problem in the community.

8.1. GENERAL RULES OF FUNDRAISING

8.1.1. Strategies for Fundraising

Having established the need for a fundraising campaign the cancer society should think of what it hopes to accomplish in its programme and consider those areas in the community where it is likely to draw most support. Fundraising can only be planned in relation to the established habits of a specific region in any country. It may be regarded rationally as a pyramid consisting of four categories in ascending order.

First Category - Fundraising among members of the public who will give donations in relation to what they earn.

Second Category - Fundraising among people with average incomes, i.e. small businessmen.

Third Category - Fundraising among professional people - doctors, solicitors, teachers, chemists, well known actors etc.

Fourth Category - Fundraising among large companies or organizations, e.g. trusts, industry, commerce, banks etc.

Obviously different methods will be required to reach each of these four groups and the following pages will deal in detail with these different methods.

In general terms, however, the cancer society must remember that it is looking for long-term support from the community and its strategy should include methods which will enable it to appeal

to the community year after year for support for its work. Despite
inflation, recession and changes in the economic fortunes of
countries, many cancer societies continue to do well simply because
their appeal is for support to help overcome the scourge of cancer.

No health problem has quite the deep emotional appeal of
cancer. It touches everyone for everyone has known someone, either
a friend or a family member who has been stricken with the disease.
Many may have seen or experienced the suffering and hardship it
brings. Some have, perhaps, had first hand experience with the
tremendous advances made by science and medicine against cancer.
This public concern about cancer is the greatest asset that the
cancer society has and its overall strategy must be based on the
concern of all members of the community to see advances in research,
successful cures and the alleviation of suffering from this disease.
Keeping these considerations before the public must be a major part
of the cancer society's fundraising publicity and is dealt with in
detail in the section on public relations.

8.1.2.   *Long-term Fundraising and Special Appeals*

Fundraising campaigns can raise anything from relatively
small to very large sums of money so the cancer society's
financial objectives will determine the type of campaign.

Whilst the Society's needs will be ongoing and will require
volunteers and groups to be steadily working away at raising funds
on a long term basis, there will from time-to-time be a need for
special 'one-time' appeals. These are campaigns to raise money
for a building or addition to a building, a special wing or
department, equipment for a department, or expensive apparatus
which is likely to be a single large undertaking requiring a
substantial sum at the one time. Such special appeals may be
named after a wel˙ known personality who has been prominent in the
fundraising campaign. Sometimes, however, it is necessary to
permit donors to pledge contributions over several years.

Careful consideration needs to be given before launching any
fundraising appeal to decide on the type of campaign. It will also
be necessary to decide on the financial target and this is dealt
with elsewhere in this section.

8.1.3.   *Cautions*

As already mentioned, great care must be taken in the fundraising appeal that the methods and message used do not conflict
with the overall message of the cancer society. Great harm may
be done by volunteers who have not been briefed and who may be
unaware of the harm that they can do the cancer society and its
work by exaggerated or inaccurate statements. (See Section *8.3.3.
Instructing Volunteers*).

8.1.4.   *Innovative Ideas*

The cancer society is working in a changing world and fundraising methods must be kept under constant review. The fundraising campaign committees of the cancer society must be always

ready to consider innovative ideas which may improve their fund-raising techniques. There are many reasons why certain voluntary organizations have been more successful than others. Some have improved their existing fundraising techniques, built up their body of regular supporters and improved their communications with them. Some have done all this and also improved in depth and breadth their understanding of actual and potential donors. They may have done this by making better use of existing information, by commissioning research or by strengthening their internal systems for recording, controlling and monitoring their fundraising and promotional programmes. Of course, others may simply have been lucky, but even luck usually comes to those who have equipped themselves to receive it. In all cases, a belief in their own cause and confidence in their quest to win support has been essential. The evidence today confirms that for any worthwhile charitable cause, the funds are available to turn ambitions into attainments if only the right measures to realise this potential are identified and pursued. Indeed, it is a potential which is too frequently under-estimated.

8.1.5. *Tax Concessions*

In many countries the state recognises the valuable function performed by voluntary bodies for the country by making some form of tax concession which is the equivalent of a financial subsidy. These tax concessions are important not only as a source of income, but also because they give status to the cancer society as a recognised voluntary organization. The system varies with different countries but the two most important are those of tax deduction and covenants.

Tax Deductions - There are various differences between different countries but the principle is the same and simple. Both individuals and firms are allowed to give a certain proportion of their income, tax free to recognised charitable organizations. In other words, if for example an American gives $100 to his cancer society, when he fills in his tax return that is put down as tax-free income. Before a tax concession of this nature is allowed the cancer society must satisfy the relevant government department that they are conducting their affairs in a satisfactory manner. Accounts and other information have to be supplied and these are closely scrutinised. Each year there must be an annual audit which will satisfy the tax authorities. However, once the society has been recognised this is in itself an assurance to the public of its bona fides, that it is properly conducted and worthy of their support.

Covenants - The main difference between the two tax relief methods of any tax deduction and covenants (which operate in Britain and some other countries) is that with the first the donor passes on the tax benefit while in the second the cancer society has to claim the tax paid. The position with covenants is that if an individual or company covenants or undertakes to pay a charity a certain sum each year for a minimum of four

years, then the charity i.e. the cancer society is able to
reclaim the standard rate of income tax payable on that
amount.   The effect of this is that if a British taxpayer
undertakes to pay say £100 per year to the cancer society
for four years, then at present rates the cancer society
can reclaim each year tax amounting to about £70.   In this
way a gift of £100 becomes £170 and over the entire period
of four years a donation of £400 becomes something like
£680.   So that as can be seen, the covenanted income
almost doubles the value of a gift to the cancer society.

8.1.6.   *Acknowledgements and Receipts*

Anyone who supports the cancer society by a donation or gift
deserves to be thanked and the way in which this is done may
determine whether or not they respond a second time when approached.
This is an opportunity to make a friend for the cancer society for
life.   If the donor has in his letter referred to any point then
a specific reply or reference must be made to that.

Modern business methods make it possible for word processors
to produce stereo-type letters which can accurately match in the
name and address for each individual subscriber.   Even so, the
letters must be personally topped and tailed with their name and
a signature of the official of the cancer society.   When large
donations are received from industry or corporations and trusts,
or when the donation is received in response to a special appeal
which has been personalised by the president or chairman of the
cancer society, then this individual would be well to sign the
letters of thanks as well.   All too often rather nondescript
replies and acknowledgements are sent which leave a poor impression
on the donor and which may well effect their decision to make
further donations to the cancer society.

An official receipt should accompany every letter which is
acknowledging donations.   This receipt should have a serial number
and be signed by the treasurer or some other official in the cancer
society.   It is vitally important that all donors be reassured
that the cancer society carries out correct accounting procedures
for all money received.   Often those making donations on behalf
of groups and other voluntary societies or commercial undertakings
will wish the letter and receipt to be placed on the noticeboard
for all to see.   This may be the one opportunity that the cancer
society has of promoting its image so that a letter heading used
on donation acknowledgements should reflect an overall image of
the cancer society, its work and objectives.

8.1.7.   *Computerised Fundraising*

The computer and micro-chip era has definitely arrived and
in this guide it is appropriate to make mention of the specialized
computerised fundraising methods currently employed by some
organizations.   This development in fundraising techniques is
widespread and requires careful planning.   All cancer societies
have a very considerable list of subscribers and potential
subscribers and it is here that computing technology can make the
task of updating and classifying these subscribers so much easier

and more efficient. Cancer societies can use computer technology with word processing facilities to open up new methods of fundraising. Computing methods offer:

- The creation of an index of regular donors.

- The selection of prospective homogeneous target groups.

- The preparation of personalised letters.

- The production of statistics plus many other advantages to the cancer society.

The days when computers were vast, expensive machines requiring a whole room to house them have long passed and the cost of a computer today should be within the range of most cancer societies' budgets.

8.1.8.   *Fundraising Consultants*

With the advent of the need for modern business methods to be used in fundraising, cancer societies may find themselves having to choose between appointing a full-time fundraising organiser to the staff or employing a special fundraising consultancy. Fundraising consultants can be employed for one-off campaigns to give general advice or retained as permanent advisers though the last is unusual. The professional firm involved will usually appoint a campaign director from among its own staff to direct the cancer society's appeal and should be able to provide back-up staff with expert advice on relevant aspects of the work, such as appeals to trusts, businesses and the preparation of publicity materials, or covenant campaigns. The calibre of such personnel and the advice that they give varies enormously from one firm of consultants to another. Unfortunately, there is no professional body to enforce even minimal standards of competence for these fundraising organizations and perhaps the high turnover in staff in these consultancies is indicative of a failure to offer the service that the firm would claim. Some disadvantages about appointing a fundraising consultant would be:

- No consultant is going to feel particularly committed to your cause since they are likely to work for many different causes and this lack of commitment will probably make the cancer society's own staff unhappy about working with them.

- Consultants will not do the actual asking for money in your fundraising appeal but will see themselves as simply in an advisory role. Often after such a campaign the cancer society may feel that it could have done better itself.

- Consultants are expensive and the society has to pay not only for its own campaign costs but also the cost of the consultant's staff time which is usually higher than the same rate paid to equivalent staff employed by the society and on top of all this the charity has to pay to cover the overheads of the fundraising consultants and leave them a profit margin.

Not all campaigns launched by professional consultancies are successful. However, there will be perhaps occasions when the cancer society does not have the personnel presently in post who

can direct their own fundraising campaign and may wish to employ
fundraising consultants for a limited period to launch a new
appeal or raise funds for a special project. In this case very
careful enquiries should be made and the recommendations of other
voluntary organizations who have used the fundraising consultancy
concerned should be obtained.

The first step then is for the cancer society to ask the firm
of consultants to draw up a proposal for a fundraising campaign
and this should be done without charge or indeed any obligation.
The proposal submitted at this stage is not likely to be final but
it will give the cancer society a chance to decide if they wish to
proceed with the next stage. Also before entering into any
contract the cancer society should ask the consultants concerned
for a list of past clients and check with them that they were
satisfied or disappointed with the results achieved. They should
also check very carefully details of the contract regarding the
costings, charges that they will be expected to cover and any
safeguards which may be offered against failure.

Good fundraising consultants can provide an efficient service
and provide the charity with much needed funds. They do charge
highly for this service however, but when their efforts are
successful no cancer society would begrudge them their fees.
Unfortunately, not all consultants are competent, therefore
great care must be taken before making any appointment.

8.2.   *ORGANIZING THE FUNDRAISING PROGRAMME*

8.2.1.   *Patrons, Committees, etc*

Every cancer society will have its own ideas about the fundraising campaign committee. The approach may differ from one
country to another; however, the following outline organization
has been tried and tested in a number of countries and works
successfully. Firstly, a prominent public figure is selected each
year to serve as campaign chairman, thus helping to draw the public's
attention to the importance of the cancer society's appeal. The
chairman assists in overcoming unforseen obstacles, initiates
contacts with institutions, industrial companies and new donors
and attracts coverage by the communications media. Suitable
chairmen might include government ministers, members of parliament,
scientists, presidents of national and industrial enterprises,
mayors and other distinguished personalities. Ideally the campaign
chairman should have executive ability and experience in organization. He must also be a leader who will attract people to work
with him through his efforts and personality. However, a good
leader is able to assign responsibilities to others so that his
committee will all be assigned their own tasks and responsibilities.
It is also important that the leader undertakes to complete the
full campaign year. He should also attract people to his committee
capable of succeeding him as leader in successive years.

Fundraising Committee - It is important that its membership be
representative of the community as a whole and should ideally
be made up of the most influential and respected citizens
available. In choosing these consideration should be given to

87

all phases of civic life. Government, professional, particularly medical, dental and nursing, industrial, commercial and representatives of trade unions, women's committees, schools, religious organizations, law, engineering, etc, as well as influential people in the theatres, arts, sport, publicity, advertising and media. This committee's influence will do much to gain the support of the community as a whole and their example should set the standard for public giving.

It is important that the campaign committee should work closely with the cancer society's full-time fundraising and administrative staff. It should complement the role of the cancer society's professional staff and through their influence should greatly widen the appeal of the cancer society to the community.

Among the responsibilities which might be given to the campaign committee will be the following:

- Enlisting campaign leaders, sub-chairman, chairman for special fundraising categories, publicity etc.

- Considering and approving comprehensive administration system of control.

- Establishing a secretariat.

- Deciding all points of policy.

- Co-ordinating all activities.

- Approving a system of financial control.

- Approving a budget for expenditure, emphasizing the importance of keeping costs down.

- Authorizing publicity programmes.

- Determining security measures.

- Ultimately to hand over all monies raised for the cancer society and make a final report.

N.B.   In some cancer societies many of these responsibilities will be given to standing committees of the organization such as the Finance and General Purpose Committee.

8.2.2.   Staff and Logistical Support

Any fundraising campaign will require staff and logistic support and the cancer society will have permanent staff whose responsibility is to provide the direction, motivation and support for the work of volunteer fundraisers throughout the country. The responsibilities of the chief executive of the cancer society will include the important task of ensuring that adequate funds are available to meet the cancer society's budgetary targets in order that its services may function properly. Responsible to the director will be the member or members of staff who have a specific responsibility for liaison with volunteers and undertaking their recruitment, training, motivation and organization.

Donations must also be the responsibility of one or more individuals who must ensure that all donations are duly receipted

and proper letters of thanks despatched promptly and the money
lodged to the central funds with adherence to proper accounting
procedures. In addition, the society must ensure that its
voluntary fundraisers are well supplied with literature, fundraising aids such as collecting boxes, flags, posters, sponsor
forms, etc.

The society must allocate adequate working space to its
fundraising staff in the headquarters with telephones available for
use by fundraising personnel. Office space allocated to the fundraising team should be convenient and accessible to volunteers,
preferably on the ground floor and with adequate area for parking
near-by so that volunteers may easily bring in returns or pick up
kits for collections. It is important to note that there must be
good liaison between the fundraising staff at headquarters and
other cancer society staff who may be employed in the public
education and information programme or in the patient care
activities since their work will often complement each others'
efforts.

8.2.3.   *Budgeting the Campaign*

As in any financial programme a budget and a timetable must
be established before the campaign is launched. Target income
goals must be set for the campaign as a whole and also for each
sub-division in the national network and regular follow-up progress
reports must be made. Comparing goals with progress will alert
the campaign committee to any areas which may need a special effort,
so that the campaign achieves its objectives. Indeed, planning is
the only way to make sure that a fundraising campaign will succeed
whether it is a one-off campaign or a continuous fundraising
programme and preparatory work is essential. This planning is
usually one of the responsibilities of the fundraising campaign
committee. They should prepare a time schedule well in advance
and distribute this so that everyone involved in the campaign
knows what is his responsibility and also the dates during which
the task is to be completed.

8.2.4.   *Publicity*

Chapter 7 on Public Relations covers in detail the methods
for obtaining publicity for all the cancer society's activities.
This applies in particular to the fundraising campaign and the
importance of co-ordinating the fundraising appeal with the cancer
society's other activities has been stressed. It will be the
responsibility of the headquarters staff to ensure that the fundraising campaign is given adequate support by appropriate publicity
and public information campaigns. Local committees and groups
operating throughout the community should also, however, be
responsible for publicity for the activities in their own areas,
contacting local journalists and media.

8.2.5.   *Fundraising Groups*

Organized groups of volunteers are the greatest asset of any
cancer society. These organize fundraising, supporting pressure
group activities, providing personnel for flag days, gain local

publicity for the society's work and all in all are the cancer
society's arm at community level. The type of organized group
can vary enormously. They can be geographically based or based
on a trade or profession. They may be specifically for young
people or for students or for either men or women only. They may
be limited to a particular school or business firm. They may be
set up as temporary ad hoc groups to deal with special fundraising
campaigns, or they may be permanent, surviving changes of membership.

     Although the cancer society can derive valuable benefit from
individual supporters in the same way as it does from its groups,
it should be recognised that groups of volunteers perform a social
function for its members and if its members find it agreeable will
sustain their interest and preparedness to help the cancer society
over many years. Since the organized voluntary group will use the
cancer society's name, care must be taken that it does not bring
it into disrepute. Therefore, the society's groups should be under
the control of the parent body and must abide by its rules and
regulations. Indeed, in some countries it is thought worthwhile
to require that each new volunteer group should register with the
society as an affiliated group and are required to complete an
affiliation form which clearly states the aims of the society. The
officers of the group are required to sign an undertaking on the
group's behalf to abide by the society's constitution. In any
case, it is important that organized groups do abide by a basic
constitution which would require the officers to be elected
annually at an annual general meeting and also that they maintain
their accounts in good order and hand monies collected over to
headquarters at regular intervals.

     Apart from overall control of these voluntary groups, it is
important to make sure that regular contact is maintained with
them to maintain motivation and to ensure that they are still
carrying out the functions which the cancer society has assigned
to them. It will require therefore that the society's staff
visit these groups on a regular basis and in many cancer societies
a group organizer is appointed with this specific responsibility.

8.2.5.1.   Formation of Groups

     Volunteer groups are formed either when someone contacts the
cancer society and says he wants to help by setting up his own
group or by a deliberate sustained canvass of the community in a
specific area with publicity to call for volunteers to help the
society's work. The following procedure should be followed when
setting up volunteer groups:

-    The group's working area should be decided whether it is to
     be geographically defined or limited by occupation. It is
     better to choose a small geographical area rather than a
     large one. If the group is to cover its chosen area
     effectively one can always establish further groups if any
     area is inadequately canvassed for funds.

-    Planning a lauching meeting. This can be held in somebody's
     home or in a public hall but the hall, in fact, should not
     be too large since it is unlikely there will be a large

audience. The venue should be convenient to public transport
and preferably a non-sectarian location. In choosing the
date try to avoid other clashing events, or even popular
television programmes, and it is usually best to arrange the
meeting so that people have time to go home after work before
attending the meeting.

- Contacting potential members. Any donors in the area whose
  names will be recorded on the cancer society's files should
  be contacted and invited to join the group being formed in
  the area and also be invited to the inaugural meeting. Local
  organizations such as rotary, youth groups and women's clubs
  and other groups should be notified of the start of the
  group.

- Publicity. Impending launch must be published as widely as
  possible. Posters advertising the meeting and the venue
  should be displayed prominently in local shops and public
  libraries up to four weeks in advance. A letter should be
  sent to local papers inviting people to join the group and
  a press release should also be issued. Announcements in
  religious meeting places and at other voluntary groups of
  the impending meeting would also be valuable.

- The Inaugural or Launching meeting. It is important that the
  cancer society personnel attending this meeting project an
  image of a lively go-ahead society with which the volunteers
  would like to be associated. If possible, show a film about
  the cancer society's work if there is one and also have a
  well-known speaker to talk about the society. There should
  be a chairman to welcome the audience, introduce and thank
  the speakers and summarise the proceedings by inviting the
  audience to join the new group being formed. The choice of
  chairman is crucial. He can make or break the meeting. He
  must be a good public speaker and be liked by the audience.
  If there is already the nucleus of a group in the area and
  the inaugural meeting is an attempt to increase numbers,
  then the chairman can invite the audience to support the
  temporary appointment of officers, chairman, secretary and
  treasurer, who will act until the members know each other
  better and then proper elections can be held.

The launching meeting should make people want to join,
enable them to do so and fire them with enthusiasm for the
work of the cancer society. The need for groups to be
affiliated to the parent body has already been mentioned.
All groups should be organized to a standard pattern. It is
usually important to elect certain of the members to serve
on a committee and undertake specific tasks.

The chairman sees that all tasks are carried out as
promised and is spokesman for the local group and chairs
meetings. The secretary notifies members of meetings, keeps
minutes, deals with correspondence and is responsible for
up-to-date lists of members. The honorary treasurer is
responsible for the group's funds and must keep an accurate
record of all expenditure and receipts and ensure that these
funds are remitted regularly to headquarters of the cancer
society. A publicity and press officer would be responsible

for producing posters, leaflets and ensuring they would be distributed, and also for sending out press notices.

All officers appointed should be active - there is no point in having figureheads as officers. If you want such people then call them 'president' and 'vice-president'. Above all ensure that you have a genial, cheerful and efficient committee, since those who enjoy their work will be successful. The fundraising committee should hold regular meetings, if possible once a month and an annual general meeting should be held by the group which will be attended by a representative from cancer society headquarters.

Once established, a group of volunteers such as this can provide financial support for the cancer society on an ongoing basis for many years provided that regular communications from headquarters keeps the group informed about the cancer society's programmes and achievements. Then the motivation will be high and there is an enormous range of fundraising activities which groups can undertake in support of the society's work.

8.2.6.   *Fundraising and Volunteers*

People who have known cancer are the first line of defence against it. They are looking for ways to fight it. They are waiting to be asked to help with their time and talents in many of the manifold tasks a volunteer organization can give them. They are, therefore, the natural first choice to raise money for a volunteer cancer association. As part of the community they can communicate most effectively with their neighbours. Although ideally they should be integrated into a volunteer group, or indeed be asked to establish their own, not everyone works well in groups and there will be many volunteers who will serve the cancer society better by working on their own. There are others too who would not have the time to give to join a regular volunteer group with its monthly programmes but would be willing to give their time on an annual basis to a one-off fundraising campaign.

The cancer society must use and channel the energy available from all these volunteers to its work and it will be the job of the campaign committee to harmonise the efforts of all volunteers, both individuals and groups, in the overall fundraising campaign programme.

8.3.   *VOLUNTEERS*

The fight against cancer concerns all, both young and old, irrespective of sex, creed, profession and social status. The task undertaken by any cancer society requires voluntary participation. Volunteers are truly the life blood of the cancer society. There is so much that they can do and there is always a shortage of hands.

Patterns of volunteer activity obviously vary in different countries. Volunteer action is more easily begun and sustained in a society where conditions favour it, i.e. where there are well organized social groups, sufficient communications and sufficient leisure time and available money. Nevertheless, it may be said that almost every society no matter what its structure and stage of development, can create important spheres of work for volunteers whether organized formally or informally. This is because volunteer activity invariably appeals to personal and social self-interest. Most volunteers' choice of organizational affiliation reflects a personal identification with the cause for which the society exists. The cured cancer patient or the person who has experienced cancer in his own family thus often proves to be the best motivated, most dedicated volunteer for a cancer society.

8.3.1.   *Recruitment*

Today many citizens with an average education, income and leisure time are both able and willing to do more than merely observe formal obligations to the community and are prepared to give both time and money to support the causes they value. Cancer society organizers must capitalise on this latent goodwill by creating a "climate of volunteering" by offering community leaders and individuals challenging and worthwhile tasks. It is very important to recruit as many members as possible who will undertake among other things:

- To participate as volunteers in one of the activities of the society.
- To give a regular annual donation and seek to participate in the fundraising and information campaigns of the society in their home town.

The recruitment of volunteers requires a variety of approaches to a great many people and these have already been discussed in the formation of fundraising groups. Some of the most obvious areas for recruiting volunteer workers for a campaign are from the following:

- Religious organizations
- Civil clubs
- Industrial associations
- Women's organizations
- Trade union organizations
- Professional groups and associations

Beyond these specific groups there will be innumerable individuals who are interested in the cancer problem. People affiliated with cancer control organizations such as hospitals, teaching schools, treatment centres, etc can be of great help. Many people in prominent positions in the community will be willing to work for the cancer cause. They must not be figureheads, but people who will take responsibility and discharge it.

The following methods have been used successfully in some countries to recruit volunteers:

8.3.1.1. *Coffee Mornings*

Invite those people who may be willing to support the work of the society. Each participant would be invited to help in two ways. Firstly, by joining the society and paying the appropriate membership fee on the spot, and secondly by organizing in their home a similar coffee morning for their circle of acquaintances who could then be asked to organize further coffee mornings for other people who would be willing to act as volunteers for the society. It is important to prepare for such meetings, not only the printed information which will be distributed, but also a definite list of activities for those who volunteer. Those who do express a willingness to help should be given some task to perform without delay when they have expressed their willingness to help, since delay often causes more harm than had no appeal been made in the first place. Wherever possible, personal contact should be maintained between new volunteers and cancer society representatives.

8.3.1.2. *Telephone Campaign*

It is possible to recruit volunteers by a special telephone campaign. This requires careful planning and preparation and it is necessary to have access to a large number of telephones in one place to be operated by a group of volunteers. They telephone the hundreds of people on prepared lists and suggest that they join the cancer society as volunteers. A business company may give permission for its telephones to be used after working hours and this permission could be accepted as a donation to the society. A list would be prepared in advance from recommendations of active local members of the community and in consultation with women's organizations, church and other groups.

The telephone campaign should be announced in advance and perhaps accompanied by radio and television publicity so that the public would be prepared to co-operate. The telephone numbers of the cancer society which individuals may phone on their own initiative should also be publicised. The team of volunteer telephonists should be trained in advance in how to make their approach. Within a few days of such a telephone campaign all those who have volunteered should be invited to a meeting with local representatives of the cancer society.

8.3.1.3. *Recruitment of Volunteers through Existing Organizations*

Another way of enlisting volunteers is by direct appeal to other community organizations requesting that they ask several of their members to work for the cancer society. The allocation of such members could be a one time effort for a particular campaign or as permanent representatives to fulfil an ongoing aim in society.

8.3.1.4. *Enlisting Volunteers for a One-time Campaign*

When an extra large force of volunteers is required for a short one-time event such as a door-knock campaign or a flag day, it is possible to turn for help to a wider range of organizations and institutions such as youth groups, university students, high school pupils, women's organizations, professional organizations, etc. In some countries it is possible to request the help of the police and government employees or employees of the local council. Senior staff members of large business concerns can also be asked to assist.

8.3.1.5. *'Ask Your Neighbour' Method*

Volunteers can also be enlisted for such campaigns by the 'ask your neighbour' method. That is to say, every existing member undertakes to bring ten extra temporary volunteers and thus fulfil the manpower requirements.

8.3.1.6. *Summary*

Every large scale recruiting campaign should be backed by an intensive publicity campaign in the local press, radio and television. Remember, when volunteers are used for a task or a fundraising campaign they should each receive a certificate or letter of thanks from the cancer society as an expression of appreciation. It is most important to keep a central register of these volunteers for further reference, listing names, addresses and telephone numbers, also professions and skills as well as the job that they have carried out in the past. A summary of the most important object-ives in using volunteers is as follows:

- Involve them in campaign planning and implementation.
- Assign them quickly to tasks which they can enjoy performing and regard as a challenge.
- Keep them informed of ongoing activities.
- Consult them and elect them to leadership posts in their local volunteer group.
- Award them appropriate recognition for their services.

8.3.2. *Motivating Volunteers*

In the long run the cancer society will be judged by its actions rather than its aims. The cancer society will most likely be involved in three essential programmes:
- Education of the public and the medical and allied professions.
- Service to the cancer patient and his family.
- Research into the fundamental nature of cancer and its methods of treatment.

How can such programmes best be combined with fundraising? Where volunteer activity can be focused on clearly defined and tangible targets, the results are likely to be better than when activity is directed solely to "general aims".

People prefer to join in concrete tasks, e.g. raise funds for the acquisition of essential but expensive medical equipment for cancer treatment, organize home services for the ill, etc. However, volunteer enthusiasm for specific projects must be tempered with the need to co-ordinate their activities in the

overall planning for it is obvious that each can contribute only
a small part of the effort needed to maintain a meaningful community
cancer control programme. The motivation necessary for volunteers
to maintain their activities for the cancer society is best
maintained by a regular flow of information to the volunteer on the
aims, activities and progress of the cancer society.

Remember that people who have known cancer are in the first
line of defence against it. They are looking for ways to fight it.
They are waiting to be asked to help with their time and talents
and many of the different tasks the volunteer cancer society can
give them. They are, therefore, the first natural choice for
fundraising for a voluntary cancer society. As part of the
community, they can communicate most effectively with their
neighbours providing they are properly instructed themselves.

8.3.3.   *Instructing Volunteers*

The greatest number of persons involved in cancer control is
the group raising funds. They should understand the cancer control
programme and be able to explain it and convey its objectives to
the public. Work for a cancer society means getting to know facts
and figures! The volunteer must also be well informed about the
society's rules, standards and policies. Volunteers should have
and be familiar with literature on all activities and programmes
related to cancer control.

Educational effort at the time of fundraising can actually
help save lives as well as create a greater interest in giving.
However, great care must be taken so as to avoid pitfalls and
controversial discussion about new and unproven methods of diagnosis
and treatment, etc. The volunteer must be careful neither to arouse
phobias nor unwarranted hopes in giving information about the
society or about cancer research and treatment. Medical questions
should never be discussed but should be referred to doctors.

Cancer society volunteers must be taught what to say when
asked about the organization and its activities. Members of the
staff of treatment centres, members of the education groups,
should present their work in detail to them so that they can
understand it and are motivated by it. Doctors, scientists and
others working in cancer research or cancer control can help
fundraising volunteers by explaining the need for funds in terms
of their work.

8.3.4.   *Fundraising through School and Youth Groups*

In many countries there is a tradition of using children as
fundraisers and a good way of fundraising in schools is where the
children can actually earn the money and where enthusiasm counts
more than parental wealth and where the children learn to be
sympathetic to the charity's cause. It is also extremely useful
in the long run to the child's education if they learn about cancer
and not simply raise money for the cancer society. Lectures to
young people at school, therefore, can have the twin beneficial
effects of increasing their knowledge about a disease which many
of their parents will regard with awe and fear, and also motivating

them to raise money to further the society's work. Usually the local education authority will be able to help by providing comprehensive lists of schools in the area or nationally.

In schools, head teachers or teachers are the key figures and it will be dependent upon their leadership and goodwill whether or not the cancer society's campaign reaches the children. The type of approach to the school will depend upon the size of the campaign to be launched but do remember when mailing to schools that a great number of other people are sending literature to them and the head teacher may respond by throwing it into the waste-paper basket, especially if it is a circular letter.

A telephone call follow-up or an individual, as opposed to a circular letter, will increase the response rate but involves a large amount of work and, therefore, staff time. As it is unlikely in the sort of mass mail out that each individual letter can be personally addressed and signed, it is often better to try and get the letter signed by a celebrity as this will greatly enhance its acceptability and interest. Remember that although it is the head teacher or perhaps youth club leader who will initially decide on whether or not to take part in the campaign, it is important that the children view the cause with enthusiasm. So try to select a celebrity attractive to both children and teachers or youth club leaders. Letters which are simply requests for money are least likely to succeed.

Generally teachers do not like to hold collections in their schools except in the case of a world disaster. The best letters are those in which the school is invited to take part in a campaign and ways of raising money are suggested. When writing to a school enclose a letter to the pupils and ask the head teacher to read it at the morning assembly. It is also useful to include a tear-off slip on the letter to the head teacher to enable them to reply promptly.

Youth clubs are a more difficult target to approach than schools because the leaders change more often and it is so hard to build up a committed body of support. Also many of these clubs will be in need of funds themselves. If you are sending a speaker into the school or club try to get someone attractive to young people. People in their twenties are generally better than those in their fifties who will seem too like the teachers. Children respond to enthusiasm and not to lecturing.

When a school or youth club agrees to help, then it helps if details and ideas for fundraising can be given and also if incentives such as badges to wear are offered. Other extremely valuable methods of fundraising among young people are competitions and sponsored events. When making contact with schools and youth groups for fundraising purposes, their attention should also be drawn to educational services offered by the cancer society.

8.3.5.   *Fundraising through Industrial Groups*

In many countries, industry has stepped into the role of the former rich patron which has been vacated by individuals since the

imposition of high taxes. Although en mass industry donates
considerable amounts to charity, the level of donations made by
individual firms is often surprisingly small. However, it is still
worthwhile canvassing industry directly for support for the cancer
society and a personal approach to the managing director or chairman of a company by a friend or acquaintance will probably be the
most successful but, of course, is not always possible. If the
cancer society cannot organize a personal approach to the company
then a letter seeking support should be sent.

As an alternative to direct support from a company the society
can suggest that it would like to talk to employees and can ask
for a notice or letter to be displayed on the employees' noticeboard and also passed through to trade union representatives
canvassing their support. It will also be worthwhile approaching
the company welfare officer or personnel officer to enlist their
assistance and arranging to talk to employees during the lunch or
other breaks during the day.

As in every aspect of fundraising, if one or two individuals
are already sympathetic to the society's work and are prepared to
be prime movers in motivating their fellow workers, this is likely
to lead to success and a small fundraising group can quickly be
established. Many firms are quite happy for their employees to
use the factory or office space to run functions after hours for
charities and others have staff and employee social clubs where
events can also take place. Some of these industrial groups can
raise quite substantial sums of money through their activities
and should have a high priority in the cancer society's volunteer
recruitment campaign.

8.3.6.   *Fundraising through Existing Community Groups*

In every society many thousands of community groups already
exist. People love to come together and join in social or
professional groupings for entertainment, for company and for
joint activities. These may be church groups, professional groups,
youth groups such as boy scouts, girl guides, trade union groups
or philanthropic organizations. The point is, they already exist
as groups with an identity of their own and although they may
often be unwilling to give long term or ongoing support to the
cancer society, they can be asked to participate in one-off
campaigns. Ideally the group will adopt the cancer society as its
cause of the year and organize a fundraising campaign on its
behalf with the society's involvement limited to providing
information on its work and collecting the cheque at the end.
However, many groups will not be prepared to be so totally
committed and the cancer society must be prepared to accept whatever support the group is prepared to bring to its cause.

8.3.6.1. *Religious Groups*

Religious groups are ideal for charity fundraising as they
have a large overall membership, are a national organization and
are usually committed to the virtues of charity. Some causes are
clearly more likely to attract church support than others. However,
cancer has a very powerful appeal for every area in the community

and the cancer society is likely to find that support is forthcoming from all the major religions in the country. As in other appeals the best way to avoid a refusal is to have a religious leader ask his colleagues on the society's behalf.

8.3.6.2. *Professional Groups*

Certain professions are likely to be sympathetic to the cancer society. Medical and nursing professional groups are an example. It will usually be possible to get the national association of a professional group to carry out 'mailing' to its members for the cancer society. It is best, once again, if the appeal is fronted, i.e. signed by a prominent member of that particular profession and it may be possible to interest the group in adopting a project for the cancer society. The advantages of directing an appeal to a professional group is that its members are usually relatively well-off and they can afford to give generously.

8.3.6.3. *Philanthropic Organizations*

Some organizations such as Rotary International, Lions, etc, have philanthropy as part of their aims. It is invaluable to a charity to win the support of these bodies, for once they have assumed a commitment they will raise funds independently and usually give substantially. Trade unions are another useful form of support for the cancer society. Individual unions give donations to a wide range of causes. (See also payroll deductions under item *8.4.2.*).

8.3.6.4. *Special Interest Groups*

Some aspects of the cancer society's work may be of interest to specific special interest groups. For instance, choral societies may be prepared to give concerts on behalf of the cancer society. Women's groups will often support the society's work which benefits women.

To summarise then, there will be many groups in the community which will provide a framework which can be used by the cancer society to reach hundreds of thousands of people. A specific campaign based upon the relevance of the cause to the group concerned or the method of raising money is important. Local groups should be asked to help with local campaigns and approaches to these groups will be more successful if endorsed by a leading member of their group.

8.4. *SPECIFIC FUNDRAISING METHODS*

8.4.1. *United Charity Funds - Trusts*

In many countries today there are a large number of charitable trusts. Thousands of such trusts date back perhaps a hundred years or more and have large or small amounts of money for specific purposes. Lists of these trusts are now available and should be consulted by cancer societies when considering their appeals. Usually the information that is contained in these directories includes the classification of charitable purposes, an alphabetical index, a classified analysis of the operation of grant making trust and an alphabetical register of grant making trusts. The advantages of such directories enable the society to select more carefully the trust most likely to support its work, rather than blindly circulating many hundreds or thousands even of such trusts with the attendant costs of such an appeal. Certainly trusts as a source of support for cancer societies are becoming more and more important as there is an increasing tendency both on the part of wealthy members of the community and industry to make their charitable contributions through such trusts with resultant tax concessions in many cases.

8.4.2.   *Pay Roll Deductions*

Pay roll deductions which are operated by some industrial organizations can produce substantial support for the cancer society. Although the amount deducted each week from the pay of employees is small, and is sometimes known as a 'penny a week' scheme, collectively the amount is a most valuable contribution to the society's work. Such schemes do require a substantial amount of organization and of course the co-operation of both the employer, the wages department who have to assume responsibility for collecting the money and the employees who have to agree that a small contribution to the cancer society is taken from their pay. Generally, such schemes are only worthwhile when done on a large scale before the costs of organizing them are recouped. However, these schemes do share the advantages of regular payments by banker's order, i.e. once people have agreed to participate they usually stay in the scheme. In France the money given by employees under the 'Franc de l'espoir' is matched by the employer.

8.4.3.   *Covenanted Subscriptions*

The nature and value of covenanted subscriptions have already been dealt with under section *8.1.6*. However, it is worthwhile mentioning the benefits of having special covenanted subscription campaigns whereby volunteers canvass their friends and neighbours with covenant forms seeking their support. Once persons have committed themselves to a covenanted donation they usually can be relied upon for support for the four year period of the covenant. Not only is the covenanted donation enhanced by the tax relief which will be repaid to the cancer society, but also it is very valuable to have a pledge of long term support for a fixed period. Often this important source of long term support is neglected by the cancer society and covenant campaigns should be a regular feature of all fundraising in those countries where they apply.

8.4.4.   *Legacies/Bequests*

Legacies are often an important source of finance especially to the longer established cancer societies. Now that wealth is more evenly distributed there seems to be an increasing tendency for people to leave something to charity in their will and indeed such bequests can grow in number with effective publicity. Legacies can form up to ten per cent or more of the total raised each year by the cancer society and will usually show an increase within four to five years of a fundraising campaign being launched. Among the steps that can be taken to encourage bequests will be to include a 'form of bequest' in appeal literature and advertisements in legal publications. It is also helpful to circulate lawyers and bank managers with copies of the society's annual report and appeal literature.

8.4.5.   *'In Memoriam' Donations*

In recent years more and more people are becoming aware that 'in memoriam' donations are a much more practical and fitting tribute to a departed loved one or friend than traditional customs of sending flowers to funerals. Many cancer societies receive very substantial donations resulting from 'in memoriam' tributes. So once again the cancer society must set out to attract such contributions by making special mention of it in their appeal literature, producing special acknowledgement cards for 'in memoriam' donations and also circulating clergy and funeral directors with details of how such donations can help the work of the cancer society. Another occasion on which such donations are received is on the annual anniversary of deaths and it goes without saying that the cancer society must be meticulous in acknowledging such donations with a suitably worded personalised letter.

8.4.6.   *Fundraising by Membership*

Many cancer societies admit members to the organization with an annual membership fee and such membership can be used to raise valuable amounts of money for the society. Members should be given a certificate or card of membership and privileges of membership should be stipulated, such as the right to vote in general meetings, annual meetings and on specific questions. Such membership can give the public the feeling that through their influence and contributions they have some voice in choosing the representatives and those who carry out the work in the cancer society.

Membership also encourages the public to follow and support the campaign and becomes a valuable source of volunteers. Many move from inactive, contributing members to being active volunteers. The cost of membership should vary for individuals, organizations and corporations. Membership fees for organizations and corporations can span more than one year and individual members should be given the opportunity of paying a suitable fee to become a 'Life' member.

8.4.7.   *Direct Mailing*

The principles and methods of direct mailing have been dealt with under the section on Public Relations. However, mention should be made here of the value of direct mail appeals for fundraising purposes. Soliciting funds by direct mail is useful in rural or remote areas, or where an organization is not yet well enough established to canvass personally. In recent years it has also become one of the means of reaching potential donors in large buildings and restricted residential areas. It should, however, be considered supplementary to the main fundraising campaign.

Any direct mail campaign requires an accurate mailing list. Careful attention to the correct spelling of names and addresses is vital. Quite apart from the list of donors which will be maintained by the cancer society, such direct mail lists can be prepared from other sources. Often a list of voters is a very useful place to start, then there are street directories, lists of clubs, etc, and telephone directories.

Experience has shown that mail solicitation raises smaller contributions from each donor than a personal appeal. It is expensive in terms of postage, maintaining lists and printing. It does, however, bring an awareness of the cancer problem to a great many people who may not be canvassed in any other way.

8.4.8.   *Door-to-door Canvassers*

The object of such a campaign is to contact every person in every house in a district community or region. The timing of such a campaign should be planned to coincide with other fundraising activities of the cancer society so that maximim publicity will benefit the canvassers. So far as possible, the canvassers for this type of fundraising should be chosen from those living in the areas where they will be canvassing.

In this sort of fundraising there is a great opportunity for passing on information about the cancer society and the canvassers can deliver important educational literature and discuss the objectives of the cancer control programme while soliciting funds.

In this, as in all activities, it is very important to involve people whose names are associated with community development such as in women's clubs, religious groups, auxiliaries and leaders and members of existing organizations. A lot of promotion can be done in advance for house-to-house or door-to-door canvassing. Radio, television and local newspapers can alert the public to the canvass and to the time that it will take place.

It should be noted that some householders will always be absent during the house-to-house canvass. These represent potential contributors who should be contacted a week or so later and it will involve the canvasser having to make repeat journeys if they are to thoroughly cover their area. People involved in such house-to-house or door-to-door canvassing must carry a certificate of authority to collect on behalf of the cancer society. Otherwise, in many countries they will be breaking the law. It is also necessary in many countries to inform local police before conducting such door-to-door collections and sometimes a special licence must be issued for the canvass to be carried out on a certain date. This is done to avoid clashing with other charities which may be collecting in the area on a specific day.

8.4.9.   *Flag Days*

A very common method of raising funds for the cancer society is by selling flags or tags on a set day. Such flags should be attractive when worn on the purchaser's clothing and should clearly indicate the cause that has been supported as well as the cancer society's symbol. When planning a flag day it is important to have enough collectors to cover a community area completely with someone at every corner of busy street intersections and volunteers to call at every home. Students and young people's organizations can often be recruited to help as flag sellers although attention should be paid to local regulations about the minimum age of young people used in such collections.

It is important to ensure that those volunteers who are collecting for the cancer society should wear identification of their status as collectors, be properly supplied with collecting boxes and an adequate supply of flags and where necessary, ensure that police permission is obtained in advance before such a flag day is organized. There should also be advance publicity and promotion of a flag day; the amount of money it is hoped to raise and how it will be spent by the cancer society. Publicity after the event to thank people who have contributed in the local press is also important.

8.4.10. *Sponsorship Schemes*

There are a wide variety of activities which can be sponsored to raise funds for the cancer society. These include sponsored walks, runs, swims, cycle rides, mountain climbs, water ski-ing, parascending, fasts, slims and so on. The list is almost endless. The great value of sponsorship is that it often involves people in an activity which they enjoy which can be used for the benefit of the cancer society.

Local schools and youth groups particularly will enjoy taking part in sponsored events. To obtain maximum benefit from their support the cancer society should supply them with the necessary material that they will need in their project such as properly printed sponsor forms and posters on which to publicise their effort. The cancer society should also arrange publicity for the event in their local press, on radio and television if possible.

8.4.11. *Marketing Activities*

In most countries, cancer societies as charities, cannot trade as their primary objective, but can do so through trading subsidiaries which can then covenant or donate their profits back to the parent body. Great care must be taken by the cancer society to have accountants examine the tax liability on trading activities so conducted, as these will differ, depending on the law from country to country. Trading of special items which can be sold by volunteers and groups on behalf of the society is however a legitimate enterprise for most cancer societies. Items to be sold may cover a wide range from Christmas cards to second hand clothes. 'Thrift' shops or 'nearly new' shops are an established method of fundraising requiring little outlay and risking no capital or very little. In this, as in any other trading ventures, confidence and business flair are important and the volunteers who intend organizing the venture must be properly advised.

Stores and boutiques have proven to be successful ongoing money raisers. Such thrift shops challenge volunteers to use their

imagination and energies. Decorations arranged for the presentation of goods give many an outlet for their talents. Experience
has shown that these shops when well organized, staffed and
managed are a success from the start and become a source of
substantial regular income. The source of merchandise is unlimited.
Appeals for new and used goods are made via radio and television,
newspaper, companies and school bulletin boards. Circulars can
be sent to special potential donors by post and direct approaches
can be made to manufacturers and distributors for rejects, seconds
and spare stock. The location of the shop is of great importance.
It must be situated in a desirable location with good visibility
in an area where there is a great deal of foot traffic and passing
trade. If possible the space should be obtained as a contribution
or at a minimal rental, but not at the sacrifice of a good location.
On some occasions it may be possible to obtain the use of business
premises where the lease has expired and is waiting for new
occupants.

8.4.12. *Lotteries*

When allowed by the law of the land, lotteries, pools, ballots
and sweepstakes have proved to be good sources for money to support
cancer societies. People are accustomed to this form of gambling
through such national lotteries such as the Irish Sweep Stake,
Quebec Lotto, Soccer Pools, Loterie Nationale, and many other sports
lotteries in different countries. Where they are permitted by
law and where they have been well organized, large and regular
sums of money have been obtained. Athletic events to which this
type of fundraising programme apply best are baseball, hockey,
football and soccer. The pay-off is based on different combinations
of single game scores and scores over a period of time.

The operation of the event is very important. The public
must be given a clear idea of the rules and purpose and must have
complete confidence that the event is honestly run from beginning
to end. The major effort goes into selling tickets for these
events. They can be sold at various outlets such as kiosks, news
stands and shops. Ticket vendors usually receive commission on
the ticket price. These are very popular gambles and there is
always a good market for tickets. The most important requirement
is to make tickets available and easy to buy. Tickets, as in any
lottery, must be numbered and accounted for within the period before
the event. Names of winners should be published as soon as the
event has concluded or the draw made and a quick presentation of
the prize to the winner made with attendant publicity.

8.4.13. *Special Events*

Often individuals who would never participate in a regular
fundraising campaign will work long and hard on a special event,
particularly if it is in their own field of interest. While
helping on a special event many learn how their talents can be used
very effectively in the fight against cancer and some will become
permanent volunteers. Even if these people never do any work again
for the cancer society they will still feel like participants and
may reflect this through generous contributions in future years.

Special events can have a great educational benefit. Literature and information reaching the public through a special event may help to change attitudes and save lives. If for no other reason, these side benefits make the staging of a special event of great importance.

Any special fundraising event organized must do two things. Firstly and most importantly, raise money - and secondly, it should enhance the reputation of the cancer society and promote its aims of conducting research, treatment and education programmes. In organizing special events there are a number of special considerations which must be borne in mind at the planning stage. These are listed below:

CHECKLIST FOR BUDGET COSTS AND PROCEDURES FOR SPECIAL FUNDRAISING
  EVENTS

Experts:	Add members to your committee who have expertise on your special problem.
Time of Year:	A temperate season - autumn or spring.
Time of Day:	Suitable for prospective attendance.
Duration:	Short or long.
Conflicts with other events:	Advance clearance with other community activities.
Space:	Engage it well in advance - School Auditorium, Civic Centre, Exhibition Hall, Gallery, National Library, Sports Arena, Theatre, TV Studio. (a) Places for boutiques of trades, specialties. Enough to allow movement of buyers and storage of extra stock. (b) Number of people to be accommodated. (c) Toilet facilities. (d) Good parking facilities. (e) Convenient transportation. (f) Supervision and security. (g) Cloakroom.
Printing:	Invitations, programmes, cloakroom stubs, posters, menus, raffle tickets, door prize stubs, directional signs, receipts.
Complimentary Ticket:	Consider the actual cost to you for each ticket, whether press or special entertainers. Keep to a minimum.
Favours, Prizes, Decorations, Costumes:	Try to get these as contributions and keep cost down to a minimum - "Money saved in expenses is money earned for your cause".
Ticket Disbursements:	Recall of unsold tickets - establish who is in control.
Taxes:	What taxes will be applicable - local, state, federal. Is tax exemption possible?
Insurance:	Make sure place is covered for accident, fire and theft. If outdoors, rain insurance etc.

Banking Arrangements:	Make in advance with a bank.
Security:	Have at least one security officer.
Cashier:	Conveniently located with adequate change.
Furniture:	Hire in advance. Allow time for bringing in, assembling and setting up.
Products:	Wrap in advance.
Prices:	Mark in advance.
Food:	What are the catering arrangements? If volunteers, you need one waiter to three tables of ten.
Liquid Refreshments:	Permits, quantities and sources. One "bartender" can serve fifty guests.
Communications:	Public address system, microphones, bulletin boards. Telephone intercom (if necessary).
Electricity:	Make sure it is adequate. Order standby equipment if likely to be needed.
Dance Floor:	90 to 120 square metres for 50 couples.
Music:	Consider cost, overtime, exact hours, bandstand requirements on public address system. Discs or tapes may do the job.
Entertainment:	Consider all costs, accommodations, transportation, housing, publicity and stage facilities for performers.
"Money Refunded"	Do not use this or similar expressions on tickets or in posters.
Commissions:	Do not offer or permit commissions to be paid on sale of tickers.
Unions:	Be sure that union labour is hired if necessary.

SPECIAL FUNDRAISING EVENTS

It would be quite impossible to summarize in this guide details of all the fundraising events which can be organized by a cancer society to raise funds. Volunteers by their own natural initiative, ideas and expertise must be relied upon to augment the following suggestions of proven events and indeed many will take pride in thinking up their own projects and carrying them out to a successful conclusion. It is right that this should be so because the challenge offered by such new ideas and projects will be one of the things which brings satisfaction to volunteer fundraisers. As a start, however, for a cancer society, the events listed in Appendix III have proven to be successful money raisers. in the past.

APPENDIX I

CONSTITUTION

The following is a suggestion for a Constitution in abbreviated format, that may be adopted by a new Organization. It will be necessary to modify the individual provisions in order to meet the requirements of the Organization and the dictates of national legislation, convention and common practice. Since this document is of such fundamental significance it is essential that it be drawn up by a lawyer who specializes in this field. Although a number of different systems of structure and organization have been mentioned in Chapter 1 it has proved necessary to select only one example for this draft Constitution. New cancer societies may find it useful to obtain copies of the Constitutions of established UICC member organizations as examples. (See page 143 for addresses.)

Article I - Name

There shall be an "(Name of Country) Cancer Society" constituted as hereinafter provided and herein called "the Society".

Article II - Objectives

The objectives of the Society shall be to develop a programme of activities to fight cancer, to foster national and international co-ordination of these activities, and to establish one national voluntary society to conduct these activities.

Article III - Functions and Powers

For the purpose of carrying out its objectives, the Society may:

(a) Approach the public at large in order to broaden its understanding and knowledge of vital aspects of cancer, such as prevention, detection and treatment.

(b) Encourage and ensure the co-operation of professional groups such as scientists, physicians and other health professionals, in the development of professional education, detection and treatment facilities, initiation of research programmes, etc.

(c) Help and assist in the treatment of cancer patients, initiate and develop welfare and rehabilitation programmes.

(d) Erect, build, repair and improve hospitals, clinics, laboratories, rehabilitation centres, early detection clinics - all in relation to cancer.

(e) Recruit and encourage volunteer groups and individuals for the advancement of the fight against cancer.

(f) Receive contributions and subscriptions, and accept donations by means of grants, gifts, bequests, or otherwise.

(g) Receive and hold lands, securities, and other real and personal property.

(h) Invest monies and hold investments, and execute any special trusts in connection with monies or property received and held by the Society.

(i) Use the capital and income from funds and property of the Society, or any part thereof, subject to such trusts, for the established objectives.

(j) Conduct any other activities and collaborate with any other organization in the attainment of the stated objectives.

Article IV - Status and Headquarters

The Society is a non-profit organization constituted in accordance with the (insert the appropriate sections of the applicable law), with headquarters located in (name of city).

Article V - Organization Structure

To accomplish the established objectives, the Society is organized into a General Assembly, Council, Executive Committees, Advisory Committees, affiliated Organizations and/or branches, officers and staff.

Article VI - Membership

Membership of a Society may be composed of individuals or of corporate bodies.

The Society shall be composed of members who shall be either:

(a) Individuals - preferably of distinction - with an interest and desire to further the fight against cancer. These individuals may possess medical or scientific qualifications in the field of cancer or may be members of the lay public. They shall be members of the General Assembly with the right to vote.

(b) Corporate Membership. Any organization or group which supports the work of the Society and whose application for membership is approved by the Council. These may also be branches of the National Society. Such Corporate Members shall elect ... representatives to the General Assembly with a right to vote. Termination of membership should be effected according to rules established by the Council. Suggested causes for termination of membership: (a) written notice of retirement provided by the member himself. (b) failure to pay membership fees. (c) disregard for the Society's regulations or for decisions accepted by its Institutions. (d) member convicted in court for a felony. (e) bankruptcy. (f) becoming of unsound mind.

Article VII - General Assembly

The management and control of the Society and the determination of its policies are vested in the General Assembly.

The General Assembly is composed of the members of the Society (or the delegates of the Organization which compose the membership).

It shall meet once a year.

The Council shall determine the time and place of meetings. A quorum shall be present to conduct the business and shall consist of ... members (or delegates of organizations) assembled in person. Each member shall have one vote and voting by proxy shall not be permitted.

The General Assembly:

(a)   shall elect the officers and members of Council, Executive and Advisory Committees, and an independent auditor.

(b)   receive reports on the activities of the Council.

(c)   discuss and approve policy programmes and Financial Reports presented.

(d)   determine annual dues.

(e)   rectify and/or amend the Constitution.

Article VIII - Council

Between meetings of the General Assembly the management and control of the Society and the determination of its policies are vested in the Council, consisting of representatives and other members, elected by the General Assembly. (The proportion of medically (or scientifically) qualified persons on the one hand and members of the lay public on the other shall be ....)

The Council shall meet not less than ... times each year, one such meeting being held at the time of the General Assembly.

The Council may delegate its powers to the Executive Committee, other Committees or Chief Executive, except:

(a)   the power to amend the Constitution and Bye-laws.

(b)   the power to fill vacancies of representatives and the power to appoint/elect the Chief Executive, Honorary members or Officers.

Article IX - Committees

a) Executive Committee

The Executive Committee shall be composed of ... persons elected by the General Assembly from its members. It is advisable to include as members of the Executive Committee Chairmen of the main Advisory Committees, the Secretary, Treasurer and Chief Executive.

The Executive Committee shall meet not less than (insert number) times each year.

A quorum shall be present to conduct the business of the Committee and shall consist of ... members assembled in person.

Each member shall have one vote and voting by proxy shall not be permitted.

The Executive Committee shall initiate programmes, policies and responsibilities between meetings of the Council, and exercise such powers as have been delegated to it by the Council.

The Executive Committee shall receive reports from the Advisory Committees and report its recommendations and decisions to the Council.

The Executive Committee may appoint such additional Assistant Secretaries or Treasurers as may be required, each of whom may be either a volunteer or staff member.

b) Standing Advisory Committees

The work of the Society is principally determined by the Committees which refer their recommendations to the Executive Committee for approval. There shall be Committees for each major programme and administrative activity of the Society of which the responsibility, size, composition and terms of reference shall be determined by action of the Executive Committee.

c) Additional Committees

The Executive Committee may from time to time designate the appointment of additional "ad hoc" and temporary committees indicating their size, appointment and nature of their responsibility to meet special problems.

Article X - Officers

The elected officers shall consist of a President, a First Vice-President, a Chairman of the Council and Executive Committee, Vice Chairman, Treasurer and Secretary General. (The Secretary General may be the Chief Executive of the Cancer Society).

(a) President and First Vice-President.
The President will represent the Society in an Honorary capacity at high-level gatherings and with key government personalities.

The First Vice-President shall act for the President in his or her absence or temporary inability to serve.

Each of these officers shall be eligible for re-election to the same office.

(b) Chairman of the Council and Executive Committee and Vice-Chairmen.
The Chairman of the Council will also serve as the Chairman of the Executive Committee and shall supervise the adminis-tration of the programmes of the Society and shall work closely with the Chief Executive. The Chairman shall preside at all meetings and provide policy and programme leadership.

It is suggested that two Vice-Chairmen of the Executive Committee be elected. Any one of the Vice-Chairmen may act for the Chairman in his absence.

Each of the above officers should represent different backgrounds:

Layman, Physician-Oncologist, Scientist.

(c)   The Secretary General.
The Secretary General shall maintain the official records of
the Society, prepare minutes of all meetings of the General
Assembly and Executive Committee, call meetings and prepare
Agendas. (In some cancer societies the Chief Executive
performs the functions and duties of Secretary General).

(d)   The Treasurer.
The Treasurer shall supervise the preparation of the (annual)
budget, make required financial reports, and supervise the
handling of the assets of the Society.

Each of the incumbents can be re-elected for two terms.
Thereafter, he may be eligible for re-election for the same
office only if he receives a majority of 3/4 and not a simple
majority as usual at the General Assembly.

Article XI - Staff

(a)   Chief Executive. The Executive Committee shall appoint an
Executive Director who shall be responsible as the chief
executive officer of the Society for the efficient and
progressive operation of the Society and for carrying out its
programmes and policies, making such long and short range
plans and recommendations to the Officers and Executive
Committee as will broaden the scope and effectiveness of the
Society. He/she shall provide continuing liaison with other
associations, regulatory and governmental bodies and others
having a mutual interest in cancer control as deemed
appropriate. He/she shall administer the affairs of the
Society to provide maximum programmes and services within
policies of the Executive Committee, and shall make a report
at each General Assembly covering the conduct of the Society's
affairs. (He/she may also carry out the duties of Secretary
General if the General Assembly so decide).

(b)   Additional staff. The Chief Executive shall appoint additional
staff within the organizational plan approved by the Executive
Committee and within approved budgeted funds.

Article XII - Funds, Audit and Fiscal Year

Funds of the Society. All monies and funds of the Society
not immediately required to be expended for the purposes of the
Society and which the Executive Committee deems proper to be
invested shall be placed in such investments as are authorized by
the laws of (insert the name of the country) for the investment
of trust funds, or as are authorized by the instrument, if any,
of gifts of such monies or funds. All other monies and funds of
the Society shall be deposited to the credit of the Society in
banks in such accounts as are approved by the Executive Committee.
Cheques may be drawn upon the Society's accounts upon the signature
of the (here insert the positions of those authorized to sign
cheques of withdrawal).

Audit of the Society. There shall be an audit of the accounts of the Society by a person duly appointed by the General Assembly who is authorized by the law of the (name of the country) to be an auditor. As soon as practicable after the end of the fiscal year of the Society, the Treasurer shall prepare and submit to the Executive Committee an audited Statement of Account exhibiting a true and correct view of the financial position of the Society at the end of the fiscal year, and transactions of the Society during the preceding twelve months' period. Such Statement, together with the Auditor's Report thereon, shall then be laid before the General Assembly.

Fiscal Year. The Fiscal Year of the Society shall commence on (insert month and day) and end on (insert month and day) in each year.

Article XIII - Annual Report

The Society shall publish as soon as practicable after the end of the fiscal year, a report of the proceedings of the Society during the period of twelve months immediately preceding the end of the fiscal year, including a copy of the audited financial statement. Copies shall be furnished to the members of the Society.

Article XIV - Execution of Agreements

All agreements required to be executed on behalf of the Society shall be deemed binding upon the Society if executed pursuant to a resolution of the Executive Committee and signed in accordance therewith.

Article XV - Constitution

The General Assembly may make, revoke, amend, vary or add to this by resolution to be passed by a majority of the voting members of the General Assembly, and providing each member of the General Assembly has been given not less than sixty days' notice in writing thereof prior to the time and place of meeting at which such action is to be moved.

APPENDIX II

UICC MODEL QUESTIONNAIRE

FOR

A HEALTH SURVEY ON CANCER CONTROL

As a step towards the encouragement of evaluation of the results of public education, the skeleton questionnaire on the following pages is offered to member agencies of the International Union Against Cancer by the Committee on Public Education.

This questionnaire, which seeks information on public attitudes and behaviour, was prepared for the UICC by Lieberman Research, Inc., in New York. It is for use by interviewers (usually professional) who have received instructions on its use: it is not in a form suitable for showing to members of the public nor is it a document for the public to complete.

It is intended to be used with a sample of perhaps 1,500 to 2,000 men and women, carefully selected to be representative of the entire population. Expert advice is vital in developing a valid population sample, and in deciding whether the sample should be limited to one city or should cover the country. Some of the questions included here may not be suitable for a particular area — and additional questions selected to suit local situations may be most useful.

The replies to such a questionnaire should offer valuable information to those planning and conducting public education programmes: if the questionnaire survey is repeated every two or three years, it will provide important data on attitude and behaviour trends.

QUESTIONNAIRE FORM

1. What do you think are the most dangerous diseases or illnesses facing people today? (CHECK AS MANY AS MENTIONED)

   Cancer . . . . □
   Dysentery . . . . □
   Heart disease . . . . □
   Malaria . . . . □
   Tuberculosis . . . . □
   Other . . . . □
   (SPECIFY)
   Don't know . . . . □

2. (a) Have you ever gone to a doctor for a complete physical check-up even though you were feeling all right?

   Yes . . □ ASK 2 (b)
   No . . □ SKIP TO QUESTION 3 (a)

   (b) Have you gone for such a check-up in the past 12 months?

   Yes . . □
   No . . □

3. (a) Have you ever had any examinations or tests to check on the possible presence of *tuberculosis or TB*?

   Yes . . □
   No . . □

   (b) Have you ever had any examinations or tests to check on the possible presence of *heart trouble*?

   Yes . . □
   No . . □

   (c) Have you ever had any examinations or tests to check on the possible presence of *cancer*?

   Yes . . □
   No . . □

4. (a) Some people have noticed something or been bothered by something which they thought might involve cancer. Have you yourself ever had anything you thought might involve cancer?

Yes . . ☐ ASK 4 (b)
No . . ☐ SKIP TO QUESTION 5

(b) Did you go to a doctor to have it checked?

Yes . . ☐ ASK 4 (c)
No . . ☐ SKIP TO QUESTION 5

(c) How long was it from the time you first noticed something to the time you went to a doctor about it?

Less than 1 month . . . . . . ☐
1 month . . . . ☐
2 months . . . . ☐
3 months . . . . ☐
4-6 months . . . . ☐
7-11 months . . . . ☐
1 year . . . . ☐
More than 1 year . . . . . . ☐

5. Would you tell me any of the signs or symptoms that may mean cancer? (CHECK AS MANY AS MENTIONED)

Unusual bleeding or discharge . . . . ☐
Indigestion or difficulty in swallowing . . . . ☐
A lump or thickening in the breast or elsewhere . . . ☐
A sore that does not heal . . . . ☐
Change in bowel or bladder habits . . . . ☐
Hoarseness or cough . . . . ☐
Change in a wart or mole . . . . ☐
Other . . . . ☐
(SPECIFY)

PRESENT CARD A

6. Here is a list of symptoms. Some are symptoms that may be first signs of cancer; others are not. Would you look through the list and tell me the *letters* of the symptoms which you think might be first signs of cancer.

A. A sudden high fever . . . . ☐
B. Unusual bleeding or discharge . . . . ☐
C. Indigestion or difficulty in swallowing . . . . . . ☐
D. A pain in the upper arm . . . . ☐
E. A lump or thickening in the breast or elsewhere . ☐
F. Nausea and vomiting . . . . ☐
G. A sore that does not heal . . . . ☐
H. Change in bowel or bladder habits . . . . ☐
I. General aches and pains . . . . ☐
J. Hoarseness or cough . . . . ☐
K. Change in a wart or mole . . . . ☐
L. A rash on the skin . . . . ☐

114

7. Here are some special tests that are often used to detect the presence of cancer. Would you look the list over a moment? (PAUSE)

   (a) Now, would you call off the letters opposite any of the tests you ever *heard of*?

   (b) Now, would you call off the letters opposite any of the tests you yourself *ever had*?

   (c) Now, would you call off the letters opposite any of these tests that you *had in the past year*?

	a. Heard of	*b.* Ever had	*c.* Had in past year
A. *X-ray test of chest* . . . . `.`	☐	☐	☐
B. *Examination of skin* (to detect the presence of skin cancer)	☐	☐	☐
C. *Digital rectal examination* (a finger examination of the rectum)	☐	☐	☐
D. *Proctoscopic examination* (an examination of the rectum made with an instrument for looking at the inside of the bowel to detect bowel cancer)	☐	☐	☐
E. *Examination of the breasts* (for lumps to detect the presence of breast cancer)	☐	☐	☐
F. *Papanicolaou test,* also called *Pap smear* or *vaginal smear test* (an examination of material from the female organs to detect the presence of cancer cells)	☐	☐	☐
None of these tests	☐	☐	☐

(NOTE: THERE SHOULD BE TWO VERSIONS OF CARD B — ONE FOR MEN AND ANOTHER FOR WOMEN. THE VERSION SHOWN TO MEN SHOULD NOT HAVE TESTS E AND F.)

8. Let's suppose you wanted to get a physical check-up that includes tests for cancer. Where would you go?

   Specialist . . . . ☐
   Doctor, own doctor . . . . . ☐
   Hospital . . . . ☐
   Cancer clinic . . . . ☐
   Other clinic . . . . ☐
   Other . . . . ☐
            (SPECIFY)
   Don't know . . . . ☐

9. Out of 100 people, about how many do you think will get cancer in their lifetime? (WRITE IN ESTIMATE)

   ....

10. If a person gets cancer, what do you think are his chances of recovering from it — a very good chance, a fairly good chance, not much chance, or no chance at all?

Very good chance . . . . . . ☐
Fairly good chance . . . . . . ☐
Not much chance . . . . . . ☐
No chance at all . . . . ☐
Don't know . . . . ☐

11. Would you be willing to work next to some-one who has cancer?

Yes . . . . . ☐
No . . . . . ☐
Don't know . ☐

12. If a person thought he might have cancer, do you think he would go to a doctor right away or would he wait?

Go right away. ☐
Would wait . . ☐
Don't know . ☐

13. Suppose that a doctor finds out a person has cancer. Should the person be told?

Yes . . . . . ☐
No . . . . . ☐
Don't know . ☐

14. As far as you know, can a person catch cancer from someone else?

Yes . . . . . ☐
No . . . . . ☐
Don't know . ☐

15. (a) Have you ever known anyone who had cancer?

Yes . . . . . ☐ ASK 15 (b)
No . . . . . ☐ SKIP TO QUES-
TION 16 (a)

(b) What happened to the person or persons? (CHECK AS MANY AS MENTIONED)

Cured . . . . ☐
Died . . . . . ☐
Don't know . ☐

16. (a) Do you smoke cigarettes?

Yes . . . . . ☐ ASK 16 (b) AND
(c)
No . . . . ☐ SKIP TO QUES-
TION 17

(b) How much do you smoke a day?

More than 1 pack . . . . . . ☐
1 pack . . . . ☐
Less than 1 pack . . . . ☐

(c) Do you smoke filter or non-filter cigarettes?

Filter . . . . ☐
Non-filter . . . . ☐
Both . . . . ☐

17. Some people think smoking is one of the causes of cancer. Others think a relationship between smoking and cancer has not really been established yet. What do you think?

Smoking is a cause of cancer . ☐
Relationship not established yet ☐
Don't know . . . . ☐

18. (a) As far as you know, are there any non-governmental organizations in this (COUNTRY / CITY) which fight cancer?

Yes . . . . . ☐ ASK 18 (b)
No . . . . . ☐ SKIP TO QUESTION 19
Don't know . ☐ SKIP TO QUESTION 19

(b) What are their names?

....

....

19. The (NAME OF CANCER ORGANIZATION) raises funds. Can you tell me some of the ways it spends money?

....

....

....

20. Do you feel the money raised by (NAME OF CANCER ORGANIZATION) is being properly used?

Yes . . . . . ☐
No . . . . . ☐
Don't know . ☐

21. Now, to complete the interview — what is your age?

24 or under . . . . ☐
25-29 . . . . ☐
30-34 . . . . ☐
35-39 . . . . ☐
40-44 . . . . ☐
45-49 . . . . ☐
50-54 . . . . ☐
55-59 . . . . ☐
60-64 . . . . ☐
65 or over . . . . . . ☐

22. What was the last grade of school you completed?

No formal education . . . ☐
Some grade school
    (1st-7th grades) . . . . ☐
Completed grade school
    (8th grade) . . . . . ☐
Some high school
    (9th-11th grades) . . . ☐
Completed high school
    (12th grade) . . . . . ☐
Some college (1-3 years) . ☐
Completed college
    (4 or more years) . . . ☐

23. Record sex of interviewee

Male . . . . ☐
Female . . . . ☐

117

```
                                    CARD A

        A.  A sudden high fever
        B.  Unusual bleeding or discharge
        C.  Indigestion or difficulty in swal-
            lowing
        D.  A pain in the upper arm
        E.  A lump or thickening in the breast
            or elsewhere
        F.  Nausea and vomiting
        G.  A sore that does not heal
        H.  Change in bowel or bladder habits
        I.  General aches and pains
        J.  Hoarseness or cough
        K.  Change in a wart or mole
        L.  A rash on the skin
```

```
            CARD B — WOMEN

A.  X-ray test of chest
B.  Examination of skin
    (to detect the presence of skin cancer)
C.  Digital rectal examination
    (a finger examination of the rectum)
D.  Proctoscopic examination
    (an examination of the rectum made
    with an instrument for looking at
    the inside of the bowel to detect
    bowel cancer)
E.  Examination of the breasts
    (for lumps to detect the presence of
    breast cancer)
F.  Papanicolaou test, also called Pap
    smear or vaginal smear test (an examina-
    tion of material from the female
    organs to detect the presence of
    cancer cells)
```

```
                CARD B — MEN

A.  X-ray test of chest

B.  Examination of skin
    (to detect the presence of skin cancer)

C.  Digital rectal examination
    (a finger examination of the rectum)

D.  Proctoscopic examination
    (an examination of the rectum made
    with an instrument for looking at
    the inside of the bowel to detect
    bowel cancer)
```

118

APPENDIX III

SOME SPECIAL FUNDRAISING EVENTS

Arts and Crafts Sales

Craftsmen who specialize in handmade jewellery, leather goods, pottery, knit goods, embroideries and local products, often need larger outlets and to become better known.

You can do them a favour and at the same time raise money for your cancer projects by holding a sale of their products.

Sales should be made in a place easily accessible, and preferably at a time of year when displays can be put in the open.

A fixed, announced percentage of the profit should go to the cancer organization which puts on the sale.

The cancer organization supplies the promotion work, publicity, volunteer cashiers and ticket sellers.

Outdoor sales of paintings by local artists can also be a showcase for the artists as well as helping the cancer cause.

These sales can produce net earnings for your cause of from £100 to £1,000, depending on the size of your event and the number of participants.

The number of volunteers who might participate would include your committee for the event, plus probably ten volunteers for ticket sales, attendance and guides.

Athletic Events

A great many athletic events in which students, amateurs and some professionals take part can be used for fund raising.

Some suggestions are: golf tournaments, horse shows, polo meets, gymkhanas, skiing events, skating contests, softball games and leagues, track meets, hockey games, baseball, football, bowling and many others.

These events are usually well attended and well supported.

To raise money on these events, the committee must organize the community and those related to the sport; parents and friends of young athletes are good supporters.

Organizing the event is the biggest responsibility for the volunteer.

These events can be counted on to raise anywhere from £100 to £2,000 depending on interest in the sport, athletic prowess of the participants, and promotion.

Auction, Silent

Donations of gifts are solicited by volunteers. The items are mainly silver, antiques, vases, lamps, china, furniture, linens, etc, by the group raising money. The major volunteer effort is in this work.

A qualified antique dealer is asked to put a minimum value on each article.

Articles and prices are then displayed alone or at a meeting or special event.

People are able to put in sealed bids on any item and for any amount up until a fixed time.

If the articles being auctioned are sufficiently attractive, each bidder can be asked to pay a small bidding fee.

At the end of the bidding time, the bids are opened and the names of the highest bidders are announced.

It is a good principle to make sure that the items being offered are workable or in usable condition.

The amount of money that can be raised varies according to the quality of the gifts being auctioned, the number of gifts, and number of those bidding.

Bridge Parties

These can be large or small. Usually the group benefiting donates tea, coffee, sandwiches and cakes. Bridge tables, cards and covers can be borrowed from various members.

Revenue for your organization will come from the sale of tickets. Tickets should admit either individuals or groups of four.

A few prizes should be available, perhaps a door prize and a table prize, preferably donated.

A decorative floral centrepiece may be donated by a florist, to go to the winner of a table.

Possible earnings from this type of event can be from £100 to £500 depending on the number attending. Volunteers organize the committee, sell tickets, run the party, and award prizes.

Balls

A Gala Ball can be very successful in raising funds in large metropolitan areas, especially where it can be related to a popular social occasion such as the opening or closing of a racing season.

Such a project requires establishing a committee - in the special case, people active in the racing field and experienced in organizing Balls.

This activity requires a large number of volunteers. Planning should start three to four months in advance.

As much as possible of the preparation and printing of programmes should be obtained locally by donation.

Attendance is by invitation only. Limiting the number of guests makes the event more attractive. Four hundred guests would be a reasonable number. Price per guest ranges from £15 to £50.

Glamourising an event with this kind of price tag requires the proper setting. It should be colourful and richly decorated, in keeping with the occasion with which it is associated. Organizing the Ball requires a Committee to secure donations of materials and to help decorate the premises; a Committee on decor and place settings; a Committee for favours; a Committee to interest young people; and the reception and dinner Committees. All the other essentials of such an event, such as catering, music, etc, must be covered as well. The dinner must be imaginative, echoing the theme of the Ball, and of a quality equalling the prestige of the affair.

Raffles can be held at the Ball to raise additional money.

Prior publicity is very important, and so is the coverage of the Ball itself. The theme of the Ball could be emphasized by having a race named for the cancer campaign.

The net proceeds for the cancer cause can total many thousands of pounds, depending on the ability of the Committee to sell tickets and obtain sponsors and donations of important articles.

"Buck" Boards

The purpose of the event is to receive contributions from customers buying drinks in bars or at soft-drink counters, and the success of the programme in each bar will depend on the man handling the forms.

The "buck" boards are about two feet by three feet in size and are of such material that slips of paper can be attached to them easily. The slips of paper are made available at the bar and are slightly larger than the £1.00 note to show the name of the donor and the slogan "My pound to fight cancer". The donor writes his name, attaches the money to the slip, and pins it to the board.

You supply the "buck" boards and the written instructions and forms showing how the event is to be handled.

This event depends on interesting bartenders or vendors of non-alcoholic drinks. It is desirable to contact local beer, liquor or soft drink distributors in your area and to discuss the plan with them.

They are usually willing to help promote this event as its simplicity and the ease with which it is handled are in part responsible for its success. Through the distributors, you will be able to contact every bar, soft-drink vendor, pub and cocktail lounge in the community.

On contacting the drink dispenser, point out that you are not asking him or the establishment to make a contribution.

The boards should be serviced regularly to make sure that they are in good condition and that, if they have been filled with contributions, they are cleared or another board is added.

The campaign should run for a short time or it will lose interest.

Three volunteers are required for each establishment to canvass for permission to put up the boards and keep them serviced.

The total amount collected will depend upon how many boards can be placed and in how many bars.

Depending on the amount of promotion prior to the event, it is possible to expect an average of £50 per board. In some instances, as much as £150 has been collected per board.

Children's Projects

Children can perform many small tasks which contribute to the cancer programme. These projects may originate at school, or in the neighbourhood, where parents may organize the children.

Some children's projects are:

1. Raking leaves, cutting grass, garden work.
2. Collecting and selling re-usable containers, paper and worthwhile salvage.
3. Collecting empty fruit baskets to resell to market gardeners.
4. Washing cars.
5. "Baby-sitting" - and possibly with pets.

Austerity Days

At schools where food is supplied to the children, they can have austerity days under medical supervision, when the meals are minimal. The savings are passed on to their favourite organization.

The amount of money raised may vary from a few pennies up to £100. This activity through the schools is also an opportunity for educational work about cancer.

Presentation of the fund should be a special occasion, such as a visit to a hospital or a research project. Publicity about a successful project is very encouraging to others.

Dances - Civic and Club

Sponsorship of dances by civic organizations, clubs or in conjunction with civic or social events for the benefit of the cancer programme can raise substantial amounts of money. The important objective is to keep the cost of the dance to a minimum. Generally 20 to 25 percent of the expected revenue is the most that should be invested in the preparation and expenses of the dance.

Music, food and bar facilities may be contributed by local organizations and firms. Various services may be obtained through contribution or sponsorship such as the orchestra, food, police guard or security, halls and publicity.

The addition of prizes, drawings, raffles, spot prizes, door prizes, interests more people in attending and adds to the proceeds.

An attendance of 400 is a reasonable objective.

The organization of a dance requires a committee with experience and good contacts with potential sponsors and contributors.

Sometimes a drink bar can be operated in conjunction with a dance. Members may sell tickets at a profit for cancer.

The amount of money that can be realized varies considerably according to the size of the community, town or neighbourhood and the quality of entertainment. Possible gross revenue, £500 or even more.

Employee Donations and Payroll Deductions

Through large companies or institutions who employ a great number of people, arrangements can be made with employees for systematic payroll deductions with the money going to cancer control.

The amount can be as low as 5 pence a week per contributor or its equivalent.

An additional advantage of the payroll deduction is that it presents an opportunity to organize meetings for employee education.

"Ghost" Employee

A variation of this was adopted in Brazil where employers listed a "ghost" employee in the name of the Cancer Society. The payroll cheque for the "ghost" employee was a contribution by the employer to the Cancer Society out of each pay period.

Since the "ghost" idea does not ask for money from employees both these plans can be used simultaneously.

Fashion Shows

A cancer group can arrange with fashion houses to sponsor a fashion show. The manufacturers furnish models to show their furs, lingerie, suits, dresses, sport clothes for various seasons, perhaps including children's and men's clothing.

Usually fashion houses and clothing stores are glad to have new audiences for their merchandise. Your group should find a fashion show an easily saleable affair.

The fashion houses will promote the show, which is usually held at a hotel, large restaurant or inn. These places, have adequate facilities for displays and a stage or promenade for models, as well as tables for breakfast, luncheon or tea.

The sponsoring organization makes its money from the sale of tickets. The price may cover merely attendance, or may include luncheon, and perhaps drinks, with a margin or profit on the food and beverages.

You, as sponsors of the event, should avoid any financial responsibility such as guaranteeing to pay for a fixed number of luncheons or cocktails, etc. Responsibility for these items should extend only to the number of actual tickets sold.

Volunteer participation is usually limited to the organizing committee and the selling of tickets.

Fashion shows will produce revenue in varying amounts, depending on the excitement of the show and the number attending. It is not unusual to earn £250 to £500 at a fashion show.

Flower or Symbol Day

Your organization could choose a flower, preferably one that is symbolic, perhaps the state or national flower, or a flower that fits into a particular season, and sell these to the public for contributions on a specific day.

On that day pretty girls with flower baskets could appear on the streets to sell flowers to passersby to carry or wear in their buttonholes.

The Flower Day has great aesthetic appeal - the charm of purchasing a flower from an attractive canvasser plus the feeling of well-being one has wearing a flower.

Spring is an ideal time for the sale of flowers because of the enthusiasm that comes to everyone with spring and a feeling of wanting to wear something bright, fresh and symbolic.

The sale of the flowers is not limited to the street. It is very important that those offering flowers for sale attain access and permission to enter shops, buildings, commercial offices and other places where people are working, as well as the official permits usually required for street selling.

It is also pleasant to sell to offices where the employees benefit from having flowers displayed.

Sales of the latter type are for bouquets and are arranged in advance. A price per bouquet is established. Delivery is made on the official Flower Day.

Flowers must be bought at a price well below that for which you will be able to sell them.

To gain the maximum "sales" it is important to find a flower that can be easily obtained - a flower that is reliable as to blooming date. If the event proves successful, future arrangements can be made with a greenhouse, florist or gardener to produce a specific quantity each year. Then it is possible to buy flowers reasonably in bulk.

This programme will involve a large number of volunteers as organizers and as sales people on the streets and in the offices. It is a pleasant, and usually successful, way to raise money.

Temporary volunteers, such as high school girls, can raise £5 to £20 each during a single day selling the flowers at busy corners, plazas and shops.

Food or Home Fair or Cake Sale

Merchandise

A Cake Sale is organized by women who make their specialities to sell in aid of some special project, usually a church project or a charity. A Food Fair is an expanded idea, including baked goods but adding gourmet foods, party entertaining and rental of boutiques which sell special products.

Boutiques could include gourmet shop specialties such as smoked meats and herb seasonings, cheeses and quality fruit, party accessories, hand-made jewellery, etc.

A fashion boutique can display outfits on members as models and take orders or sell there. They may give 10 percent on future sales in a limited period, but naturally must be a trustworthy shop.

Baking tables of course include the usual breads, cakes, desserts, casseroles, cookies, jams, jellies and pickles. It is wise to wrap all food ahead of time in plastic sheet and mark prices clearly.

Time and Place

In a northern climate, the best months are October and May. In a large urban community, it is not too much to expect 1,000 persons to come. A Cake Sale should be held in a residential or suburban area and the hours should be short, such as 11.00 am to 2.00 pm. Most of the people will come early. For a Food Fair, the hours will be longer, such as 1.00 pm to 10.00 pm as the rented boutiques take time to set up and the larger quantity of merchandise brought in takes more time to sell.

The rooms where the sale is held should be large enough for long tables to display goods, with space behind these for storing and display, keeping boxes and bags, and for a cashier. A school or church auditorium or civic centre is the usual choice, and often has to be engaged months in advance.

Rent, Parking, Transportation

Rental of place should include clean-up before and after, electricity, tables and chairs as needed, and access the night before.

Good parking facilities and convenient transportation are essential in a large community. If it is a large affair, police are needed for traffic control, security officers to watch the cash and banking and a first aid station just in case of need. Insurance should be carried for accidents but public places are usually covered by the proper insurance. If held partly outdoors, consider rain insurance. This is costly and its value must be weighed carefully.

The rent charged to boutiques should be calculated on the interest and excitement they add and the customers' cash they subtract. It is good advertising for them and a selling point for the Food Fair.

In some cases where the sponsoring group is well known for the quality of its baking and presentations, tickets can be sold by its members in advance. These usually cover the rent and assure attendance at the sale. Door prizes can be solicited from firms to add incentive to attending the sale.

Checkroom, Bar

A checkroom is a great asset, to leave people's hands free to do further shopping, to raise money in checking fees, through the sale of shopping bags.

At an evening Food Fair a bar is a good moneymaker. Also it gives the affair a festive air. Free coffee or tea can be offered in the afternoon as a special gesture.

Decor

It is attractive to decorate, in a unified theme of colour or symbols, tables, backgrounds, wearing aprons, etc, identifying the name of the group.

Competing table settings on various themes can be spread between the baking tables, to attract interest, but must be guarded constantly.

Commerce and Banking

Food demonstrations can be set up by gas companies, meat or food companies or by famous cooks doing their specialty, etc.

Banking arrangements are essential. It is wise to have a cashier for each table who gets her original change from one Treasurer and returns her proceeds to her. This gives a check on the value of each section. The Treasurer should have extra change at hand and several assistants as "runners" and for checking in at closing time. All banking arrangements should be made in advance with bank and security officer.

Attendance - 1,000. Total Income - £5,000. Net - £3,500.

Other Activities at the Same Time

Antique sales - either auctions or rental of space to dealers.
Rummage sales - sale of used books (good but heavy to handle).
Auctions of donated items (good in small groups).
Bingo Parties (licence needed).
Cocktail Bar (with or without dancing).
Lotteries (tickets sold for art work or for cash).
Raffles - for donated articles of value.
Restaurants - offering a dinner for two as advertisement.

Volunteers

A Food Fair will require many volunteers. First are those who will undertake to supply various types of food, cakes, casseroles, bread, sauces, etc.

Next, are all those responsible for collecting the food and arranging it for sale.

Then, volunteers for decorations, checkrooms, cashiers, etc.

Fountain or Handy Receptacles in Public Places and Stores

The idea of the public fountain into which coins may be tossed for "good luck" is perennially attractive.

If possible the fountain should be where it is always under supervision to safeguard the money : inside buildings or in parks, or in much used public places.

An extension of this idea is to have small receptacles, either glass or plastic, near the cashiers in restaurants, shopping centres, banks or stores - anywhere where people handle small change and may drop a few coins in handy containers.

Receptacles and coin boxes should be attractive, colourful, and well marked with the name of your organization. They should be placed where they are readily seen, rugged in construction, and strong enough to contain the weight of many coins. A broken container is very bothersome to the cashier, storekeeper or store manager.

Fountains and receptacles require regular servicing by members of your organization because when a container is full, no more gifts are made. Also, there is the danger of it being broken and the coins lost.

To ask storekeepers to service or let a coin receptacle stand on the counter year round is asking too much.

While the fountain can be available year round in temperate climates, the coin boxes and receptacles work best when restricted to a certain period, perhaps one month, when prominence can be given to them.

A coin receptacle can accumulate from £10.00 to £25.00 within a month's time.

This project would take a considerable number of volunteers, both to place the containers and to service them.

Garage, Attic and Yard Sales

Garage sales, attic sales, yard sales, rummage sales, used clothes sales, and "white elephant" sales - all appeal to people's interest in browsing and looking for rare bargains.

The sale usually takes place in the spring, on one day (with an alternate rain date), from early in the morning until closing time.

Prior to the sale, the Committee accumulates miscellaneous items from people who are renovating their homes, moving or disposing of surplus. Articles for sale can include garden tools, furniture, oil paintings, luggage, clocks, appliances, musical instruments, and all sorts of wearing apparel and household articles.

Clothes are best displayed on racks; assorted dishes and household articles should be piled on tables.

The event should be well publicised in advance. The cancer programme which it is supporting should be well advertised in the press, on the radio and on television. This is a key to the success of such a sale, informing the public that it is for the support of cancer programmes.

This event depends on the ingenuity of the committee sponsoring it. It also depends on the number of usable articles in good condition available. It is very important that the merchandise does not appear as "junk".

These sales require very little investment as most of the items are contributed; which means that proceeds are almost pure profit for the cancer programme.

Such sales can earn £100 to £500. A really large one in an auditorium, stadium, hall, etc can earn several thousand pounds.

There is need for many volunteers to collect articles from donors, arrange them for the day of sale, and to act as cashiers, guides and attendants.

Greeting Card Sales

The sale of greeting cards, calendars, book marks, etc for a holiday or festival, such as New Year's or many religious holidays, can be very profitable.

Try to interest a printer who can supply the items at a price that will leave a margin of profit for your organization. Or go to one of the large manufacturers who has national distribution.

The price at which you sell must not be greater than that charged by other sources of supply.

This can sometimes be achieved by asking printers to do the work during the slack time of the year, or buying last year's overstock from manufacturers.

It is important to understand and know the kind of merchandise that is available, and it is also important that you choose designs that will be distinctive and carry your organization's message as well as a greeting for those who are sending the cards. Give a choice of several designs. Offer them in packages of tens or more.

A footnote is desirable, preferably in fine print, to the effect that "The proceeds from the sale of this card will be devoted to the fight against cancer".

Orders for the cards can be solicited many weeks in advance.

Members of your organization, particularly those charged with the responsibility for the venture, should canvass all their friends, organizations and industrial groups well in advance to assure that the proper quantity is ordered.

Commercial and industrial organizations are good prospects for these cards. They often use such cards in greetings to their customers or associates and are proud to show they have made a gift to your cause.

The sale of cards, calendars, etc can easily become an annual event; and a committee to arrange the preparation and to handle the details could carry on throughout the year. This can produce a regular annual income.

House of Cards

This is a programme for raising a specific sum to purchase equipment, build an addition or equip a whole wing of a hospital or clinic.

The procedure is to draw on a great number of cards, pictures of the particular items needed indicating the cost of each so that a person can donate the price of one or more items. These can include small instruments, equipment or parts of equipment, windows, doors, walls, rooms or wings of a building.

The potential donors are shown the cards at a reception given by a prominent citizen, preferably someone involved in the cancer programme - such as a director of your organization, the head of a research or treatment centre. Donors may purchase the cards then and the purchased cards are put together to build "a house of cards".

After the initial event and announcement, other prospective donors, individuals or corporations, should be visited by your most prominent members.

Plaques may be placed on important items after they are installed, to show who the donors were.

Personal Contributions in Kind

Even people who do not normally have money or cash available may make regular contributions to the cancer cause from their own produce, supplies or staple foods.

For instance, a cup of rice, basket of potatoes, a pound of coffee, ears of corn, fruit, cans, jellies; all of these may be taken to a headquarters to be sold through auctions, fairs or otherwise.

This is a very satisfying method of permitting a great many people who do not have much cash to donate.

The organization of this event is patterned after that of a food fair.

Memorials - Memorabilia

In the case of a bereavement, many people will respond to a request to give money to a worthy cause, rather than sending flowers.

Many cancer organizations have established the custom of accepting such gifts. When a gift is made, your organization should send a proper and suitable card to the bereaved saying that the person named on the card has made a contribution to the cancer programme in memoriam to the deceased, whose name is shown. The card shows the name of the donor but not the amount of money. The amount of the gift in money is acknowledged only to the donor.

This can become a very sizable source of funds and, if established as a custom, continue to bring in contributions regularly.

Gifts in memoriam need not be made only at the time of a funeral, but can be given later as a memorial to a person or persons who have departed and whose names the donor would like to have perpetuated.

Some organizations have prepared re-usable artificial flowers and wreaths for use at funerals which carry the emblem of the Cancer Society and indicate that a contribution has been made to the cancer programme.

This programme of memorials requires a location accessible to the bereaved family or friends of the deceased where they may easily make arrangement; or a method of doing so by telephone.

Funeral homes can be contacted and arrangements made to leave in their parlours a supply of cards which can be filled out at the time of visits to the funeral home for memorial donations to cancer.

Sometimes the funeral director or a member of his office staff will collect the money and issue receipts on behalf of the cancer programme, regularly remitting the money.

Merchandising Plans

A. *Commerical Stores and Restaurants* - may be persuaded to give the profit of one day's business to the cancer control programme, or to a research project or another purpose. The day or event is publicly advertised and members of the local cancer organization take it upon themselves to urge as many people as possible to buy on that day because of the benefits to cancer control.

This plan can be based on the profits for the day, a percentage of the total sales for the day, or any basis agreed on with the establishment participating in the plan.

B. *Booths or Stalls at Market Places* - A regular booth at local markets or festivals may be identified with your organization. The public can become accustomed to finding bargains there which leave a profit for the Society.

These booths or stalls can have their sales augmented by contributions from the members of home-grown produce, home baked or canned goods.

Movie Premiere

A local theatre may be induced to set aside the opening night of a first run movie for the benefit of cancer control.

The cancer programme may receive the total revenue of the first night or a premium on special tickets for traditional "first night" attendance. Generally there is no expense to the cancer programme.

The success of a benefit premiere depends on publicising the philanthropic purpose, as well as the movie itself. If possible, personalities in the film should be encouraged to be present at the time of the opening.

Press, radio and television coverage of the opening night can create much valuable publicity for your organization.

The premiere of a movie offers a lot of opportunities for imagination to create a festive and successful occasion. There are many possibilities for special pre- or post-theatre parties at even greater premium prices. Attendance at these parties by stars of the film could make them even more attractive.

Speakers and Entertainers

Your organization can invite prominent people in civic, religious, technical or medical fields to speak to groups. They can come as a panel, with a moderator to distribute questions or topics, or as individuals.

They can speak on your cancer programme on their travels, interesting activities or on historical matters.

Prominent entertainers or actors may be persuaded to give a special performance for the benefit of the organization.

On these occasions your organization should sell tickets, preferably in advance, clearly indicating that cancer control is the beneficiary, as well as promotional information on those speaking or performing.

Professional speakers and entertainers may consent to appear at a benefit on the occasion of their making an unexpected visit to your community. If there has not been time to sell tickets in advance a collection can be taken at the door or among the audience.

There is a great educational opportunity when prominent medical men discuss cancer and answer questions from the audience. These events, and the discussions and statements of the medical participants, are good copy for all the news media and will help your educational objectives as well as raise money.

Parties

Receptions and parties on some special occasion are a very popular way of raising money. A cancer group could, for example, sponsor the opening of a new public building, a museum, art gallery, a science centre, municipal buildings, and so forth. Many donations or partial donations can be made by various sponsors. Important donations are : a place in which to hold the event; a supply of food, liquor or wine or other beverages that will be sold or given to each one paying admission.

A friend of the cancer programme might offer an attractive home or garden for the occasion. It would have to be spacious enough to accommodate the crowd that would attend. This may attract many who might not otherwise have the opportunity to visit the place.

Another variation is to stage a party in an embassy or a trade commissioner's office of a country willing to supply a national specialty such as wine, cheese or other items. This creates excitement and interest in attending the function. Sending invitations in advance adds to the prestige of attending.

Generally it is desirable to charge an admission fee as well as sell drinks and food.

It is often useful to offer entertainment or music to add excitement and interest, and to justify the admission fee.

The volunteer organization will be the Party Committee - attractive lady cashiers to sell drink tickets and volunteers to pass hors d'oeuvres.

A committee to select names of invitees and send personally addressed invitations is recommended. A publicity committee or specialist can be very useful.

Profits come from admission, and sale of drinks. They can range from £250 to £1,500 or more.

Raffles

A raffle usually offers a desirable prize or prizes, such as airplane flight holiday, an automobile, a boat, a colour TV set, a new house or other wanted objects that would induce a great number of people to purchase chances.

The object of the raffle is to sell enough tickets to cover the cost of the prizes and tickets and to obtain a surplus for the cancer project.

If possible, of course, the prizes should be obtained as a donation.

A successful raffle requires selling a lot of tickets, and this requires a lot of ticket sellers. The organization of the sales programme is very important.

Every member of the organization or committee should take the responsibility of selling a minimum number of tickets. Raffle and lottery tickets are easy to sell, but it is necessary to give people a chance to know about them and have them available.

Non-members, too, may be encouraged to sell books of tickets, containing five, ten, fifteen or twenty tickets; and be given either one free ticket for every ten sold or some similar incentive.

This gives even a wider distribution and a much larger sum to work with.

Experienced promotors or public relations people should be asked to assist in the planning and the promotion.

A successful raffle requires a great many volunteers. The expenses involved are the cost of prizes, if they cannot be obtained as gifts, and the cost of printing the tickets and posters.

Lotteries, "Pools", Sweepstakes

Lotteries, pools and sweepstakes have proven good sources for money to support cancer programmes.

People are accustomed to this form of gambling through the Irish sweepstakes, the Quebec "Loto", soccer pools and sports "totos" in many countries.

Where they are permitted, and where they have been well organized, large and regular sums of money have been obtained.

Athletic events to which this type of fund raising programmes apply best are baseball, hockey, football and soccer.

The payoff is based on different combinations of single game scores or scores over a period of time.

The operation of the event is very important. The public must be given a clear idea of the rules and purposes; and must have complete confidence that the event is honestly run from beginning to end.

The major effort goes into selling tickets for these events. They are sold at various handy stations such as kiosks, news stands, drugstores. Ticket vendors receive a commission on the ticket price. These are very popular gambles and there is always a good market for tickets. The most important requirement is to make the tickets available and easy to buy.

Tickets, as in any sweepstake, must be numbered and accounted for within the period before the event. Names of winners should be published as soon as the event has concluded, and quick public payment made.

Stickers and Imprints

Your organization may arrange with a manufacturer of a standard product to have it specially packaged with an imprint indicating that you are selling it and receiving a percentage of the price.

Some items sold this way are toothbrushes, pencils, pens, brushes, etc.

It is sometimes possible for package imprints to indicate that you have been given a special privilege by the manufacturer.

This is a type of activity that should be, like a tag day, organized to be completed within one day.

It requires a very great number of canvassers who are on the street where crowds gather.

Sometimes a local service club such as Rotary, Lions or students will take the responsibility to sell on every corner and to visit houses as their contribution to cancer control.

TV and Radio Telethons

A programme director of a television or radio station may be sold on the audience value and public relations usefulness of this programme, on which cured cancer patients, students, sportsmen, research workers, medical people are interviewed on cancer by prominent disc jockeys and local entertainers.

A telethon usually goes for a number of hours, perhaps as many as twenty-four.

It is important to have continuous and interesting interviews and a good interviewer. After each interview or event the interviewer asks the listeners or viewers to send in pledges of money.

The interviewers can make appeals in their particular fields. For instance, a research worker can stress the importance of money for research. Cured cancer patients can speak about the need for money for educational work to save more lives and for rehabilitation.

The enthusiasm created by disc jockey interviewers is very important. They should continually report the amount of money raised, give the names of donors and perhaps play requested music albums or taped or telephone interviews with famous people.

Depending on the area covered by the station, substantial money can be raised : in a smaller community £500 or £1,000 up to many thousands in the metropolitan areas.

An additional feature of such programmes is the auctioning during the programme of records accumulated by the stations. They acquire a very large number of these, which have "conversation piece" value to those who buy them.

Flag or Tag Days

A very common method for raising funds is by selling tags on a specific day.

Tags should be attractive when worn on the person's dress or costume and should clearly indicate the cause that is being supported as well as your trademark.

The objective of a tag day is to have enough solicitors to cover a community completely, with someone on every corner of the busy intersections, and volunteers to call at every home. Students or young people's organizations can be recruited to act as "taggers".

It is very desirable that this be done all in one day which in itself focuses attention on its purpose.

It also makes it more important to each potential purchaser that he should be wearing a tag as others are doing.

There should be advance publicity and promotion of a tag day, its reason, the amount of money it is hoped to raise, and how it will be spent.

Special Taxes or Postal Stamps

Many countries or states have authorised the imposition of a special tax on the sale of cigarettes and other tobacco products. The proceeds of this tax go exclusively to support cancer research or for the construction of hospitals.

To establish such a tax the government must be persuaded of the vital importance of cancer research.

Some countries have authorised a postage stamp dedicated to the fight against cancer.

The sale of this stamp could be restricted to the annual campaign period.

The stamp need not be a revenue-producing stamp for the postal system. It could be an extra "seal" in recognition of the cause. The price of the seal may be set at the option of the user.

The seal could commemorate the cancer campaign, if it is an annual event.

Tours

A home or garden tour is very popular with women, particularly those interested in interior decorating, art, architecture and garden planning. Several estates, either with beautiful gardens or lovely houses, may be opened to the public on specified days. The locations of the houses and gardens are given in the invitation with a map so that they can be easily located. Admissions are sold in advance as well as at the doors of each place.

In a garden or home tour, it is advisable to have a large number of volunteers acting as attendants to direct visitors and look after valuable flowers or furniture, and to check tickets. If there is valuable art, a guard may have to be hired.

All of the places should be easily accessible by normal transportation, or special transportation should be arranged in advance.

The earnings from such an event vary considerably. If it is a one-day affair, it is possible to earn £500 to £1,000. If it is spread over a weekend the earnings may be even higher.

As indicated, a large number of volunteers would be required to participate - probably 50 or more depending on the size of the estates and gardens.

Thrift Shops

Stores and boutiques have proven to be successful ongoing "money raisers". These "thrift shops" challenge volunteers to use their imagination and energies. Decorations, arrangement and presentation of goods give many an outlet for their talents.

Experience has shown that these shops, when well organized, staffed and managed, are a success from the start; and become a source of substantial, regular income.

The source of merchandise is unlimited. Appeals for new and used goods are made via radio, television, newspapers, company and school bulletin boards, etc.

Notices and pledge cards are sent to special potential donors.

Direct approaches are made to manufacturers and distributors for rejects, seconds and overstock.

Location of the shop is of great importance. It must be situated in a desirable location with good visibility in an area where there is a great deal of foot traffic.

If possible, the space should be obtained as a contribution or at a minimum rental, but not at the sacrifice or a good location.

The organization of a thrift shop starts with a committee which establishes the operating policies, chooses the location, advises on banking and sources of merchandise and sales promotion.

There very likely should be an additional committee called the "steering committee" composed of those volunteers who have major responsibilities in the operation of the shop. For instance, there should be people responsible for the following:

(a)   Personnel
(b)   Pricing
(c)   Sales Promotion
(d)   Shop Decor and Maintenance
(e)   Merchandising

All of these key people will have special responsibilities, indicated by their titles.

The personnel director is responsible for the assignment of the working hours to the volunteers. She makes sure that there is an adequate reserve of help and talent.

The pricing director should establish reasonable prices for the merchandise. Her assistants should research the current prices for various items. They should, if possible, have some background in pricing, making up labels, giving discounts and, above all, knowing when merchandise should be thrown out.

The sales promotion chief should plan what items should be put on sale, which should be displayed more prominently, and which should be put away for other seasons. She should also be concerned with the publicity and contact with organizations that might be potential buyers.

Maintenance is very important. The shop should be neat and clean. This is even more important when used, donated or reject material is being offered for sale. And much attention should be paid to being sure goods are presented attractively in the best possible condition, cleaned and usable.

Merchandising - fresh merchandise must flow constantly into a thrift shop. It differs from a retail shop where stock can be ordered regularly. Needless to say, it takes a great deal of ingenuity to find sources of supply for additional material. A large number of volunteers are needed to make contacts and search for material to sell.

All the members of the cancer organization should be advised by cards regularly of the need for merchandise. It is very important that the goods be in style, and in saleable condition.

Some of the merchandise interesting for thrift shops is children's clothing, women's clothing, men's clothing, bric-a-brac, linens, shoes, books, jewellery and toys.

Again it is worth repeating that thrift shops have been very successful in bringing in money and involving volunteers.

They are also good places for cancer education and for diplaying the activities of the cancer society.

Thrift shops with a reasonable revenue or a turnover of sales find that their costs run about 10 percent of their income. This means that every £1.00 of sales means 90 pence profit for cancer.

This project has no barriers or limitations geographically or population-wise. Regardless of location, proper planning and operation will ensure the success of the shop and bring in sales, volunteers, and visibility for your cancer programme.

Trend Teas

"Trend teas" are a series of teas. The organizing committee puts on the first one and invites a group of ten people. These ten pay for the tea in an amount established in advance, perhaps £1.00 per person, or through a silver collection. Tea, sandwiches and cookies are supplied by the committee.

Each of those attending the meeting then forms a tea committee of his own and invites ten people. The procedure is the same, with these guests returning to organize teas of their own.

This pyramiding of teas reaches a great many people and becomes a good forum for cancer education as well as a means of raising funds. At each tea some cancer subject, or event, of interest should be presented by a prominent speaker - a research worker, a doctor, a cured patient, or someone well informed on the topics of the day.

Walkathon (Sponsored Walks)

A Walkathon is one of a group of community "action" events in which a great number of people can take part. Other similar ones are bikathons, swimathons, etc.

These events are usually organized by an adult group as there is a great deal of planning and money involved. Frequently the participants are in the highschool, teenage or younger areas.

Sundays and holidays have proven to be the best days for this event. The local police and traffic control should be alerted and their co-operation solicited.

Prior to the event, those expecting to participate are given cards which they ask sponsors to fill out. The sponsor may choose an individual participant at so much per mile - one pence, twenty five pence, a pound, and so on.

During the event the participant has a card on which his passing each station is recorded. At the end of the event he is given a certificate that shows the distance he has travelled, and then he returns to the sponsors to collect the money (the amount per mile agreed on times the number of miles travelled).

The event can be very interesting to the public and with proper promotion in advance a great number of people will turn out to cheer the participants, particularly if they have friends or relatives in the event.

At intervals the organization conducting the event will have tables or stands set up to supply water, perhaps sandwiches, and first aid for any requiring attention during the event. These stations also provide a meeting place for parents to pick up their children or to receive messages.

This type of event has raised substantial amounts of money. The cause for which the money is being raised influences the type of attendance and sponsorship.

Some local community projects where a single school or club has participated have raised a few hundred pounds and up.

Where the event has been for a hospital or a cause of deep concern to the public, many thousands of people may turn out to watch and to sponsor, and the earnings can reach £10,000 to £20,000.

The promotion of these events determines to a great extent how well they are attended and sponsored, although the sponsors are obtained by the participants. The latter are a very important factor in the success of the programme.

In organizing such an event, the number of people involved in assistance and management can total up to 125.

If the event covers a long distance, more stations will be required, all of which should be manned by two or three persons.

Similar events are:

Swim-a-thon - would take place in a large swimming pool or in a lake or river, but would certainly not cover as large an area, and generally with younger participants.

Bikathon - using colourful two-wheel bicycles, and participants of all ages.

Skatathon.

Rockathon.

These types of events are easily organized for they do not require large investments by the sponsors; and a great many people participate and enjoy having made a contribution.

"Wish for a Cure"

A variation of the fountain or receptacles for contributions is a project called "Wish for a Cure" for cancer.

A local shop may be persuaded to place a wishingwell in a prominent place where many may see the action, the money in the well, and respond to the idea : tossing a coin for a cure for cancer.

On the occasion of their making a "wish", they may also guess the total amount of money that will be in the wishing well on the closing date, which can be the day the cancer campaign ends.

A maximum amount is set for the prize, and a local merchant may agree to donate merchandise. The value of the merchandise will not be in excess of the amount established in advance.

APPENDIX IV

LIST OF UICC MEMBER ORGANIZATIONS

236 Member Organizations in 80 countries

Algeria *

Prof. A. Yaker
Société Algérienne de Pathologie
Laboratoire Central d'Anatomie
Pathologique et de Cytologie
C.H.U. Mustapha
Alger / Algérie

Argentina

Dr. Abel N. Canonico (President)
Asociacion Argentina del Cancer
(ASARCA)
Tucuman 731
Buenos Aires 1049/ Argentina

Asociacion Argentina de Oncologia Clinica
Hospital Militar Central   .Clinica
Luis M. Campos 726-7o piso
Buenos Aires 1426/ Argentina

Mrs. Ana Maria Basone de Ludmer
(General Secretary)
Centro de Educacion de las
Enfermedades de la Mama (CELAM)
Avenida Pueyrredon 1361
Piso 9"A"
Buenos Aires 1118/ Argentina

Dr. Roberto A. Estévez
Oncology Department
Del Salvador University
Av. Santa Fe 5089 - 9o piso
Buenos Aires 1425/ Argentina

Mrs. Lucrecia Travers de Williams
(President)
Direccion Argentina Filantropico
Asistancial de Citologia
del Cancer (DAFACC)
Larrea 970
Buenos Aires 1117/ Argentina

Dr. José Maria Mainetti (President)
Escuela de Oncologia de la
Provincia de Buenos Aires
Fundacion José Maria Mainetti
8 No. 706
La Plata 1900/ Argentina

Dr. Eduardo A.M. Dominguez (Director)
Hospital Municipal de Oncologia
Patricias Argentinas 750
Buenos Aires 1405/ Argentina

Dr. F. Celeste (Director)
Instituto de Oncologia
"Angel H. Roffo"
Universidad de Buenos Aires
Facultad de Ciencias Médicas
Avenida San Martin 5481
Buenos Aires 1417/ Argentina

Prof. Dr. Clemente J.L. Morel
(Director)
Instituto de Perfeccionamiento
Médica Quirurgico
"Prof.Dr. José M.Jorge"- I.P.M.Q.
Hospital de Clinicas
Cordoba 2351
Buenos Aires 1120/ Argentina

Sra. Martha de Tomasi de Gonsalez Vidal(Prsdt)
Liga Argentina de Lucha contra el Cancer
Araoz 2380
Buenos Aires 1425/ Argentina

Mrs. S.R.G. de LLorens Herrera (President)
Liga Popular de Lucha
contra el Cancer
Diagonal 74 no.1578
La Plata 1900/ Argentina

Dr. D.L. Perazzo (President)
Sociedad Argentina de Cancerologia
Av. Santa Fé 1171
Buenos Aires 1059/ Argentina

Australia

Mr. L.A. Wright (Executive Director)
Australian Cancer Society
P.O. Box 4708 GPO
Sydney, N.S.W. 2001
Australia

Miss Adrienne Holzer (Secretary)
Anti-Cancer Council of Victoria
90 Jolimont Street
East Melbourne, Victoria 3002

Australia

Dr. Peter Cooper (Chairman)
Australian Capital Territory
Cancer Society, Inc.
P.O. Box 135
Civic Square
Canberra, A.C.T. 2608
Australia

Mrs. C. Deverall
(Acting Executive Officer)
Cancer Council of Western Australia
184 St. George's terrace
Perth, Western Australia 6000

Mr. L.J.Baillie
(Hon. Secretary/Treasurer)
Tasmanian Cancer Committe
G.P.O. Box 191 B
Hobart, Tasmania 7001 / Australia

Mr. T.R. Osborn (Secretary)
The Anti-Cancer Foundation of
the Universities of South Australia
G.P.O. Box no. 498
Adelaide, South Australia 5001

Mr. John Smith (Secretary)
The New South Wales
State Cancer Council
G.P.O. Box 7070
Sydney, N.S.W. 2001/ Australia

Mr. W.L.Rudder (Secretary)
The Queensland Cancer Fund
P.O. Box 201, Spring Hill
North-Birsbane, Queensland 4000

Australia

Mr. G.S. Bolitho
(Chief Executive Officer)
Cancer Institute (Peter MacCallum Hospital)
481 Lt. Lonsdale Street
Melbourne, Victoria 3000

Australia

Austria

Bundesministerium für Gesundheit
und Umweltschutz
Stubenring 1
1010 Vienna / Austria

Prof. Dr. Hugo Husslein (President)
Oesterreichische Krebsliga
Spitalgasse 23
1090 Vienna / Austria

Belgium

Prof. C.Gompel
(Secretary General)
Oeuvre Belge du Cancer
21, rue des Deux-Eglises
1040 Brussels / Belgium

Bolivia

Senora Doris A. de Howson
(President)
Fundacion Boliviana contra el Cancer
Casilla de Correo 1406
La Paz / Bolivia

Dr. Rubén Dario Urey (President)
Sociedad Boliviana de Cancerologia
Instituto Oncologico del
Oriente Boliviano
Casilla 1265
Santa Cruz de la Sierra

Bolivia

Brazil

Dr. Jorge de Marsillac
(President)
Associaçao Brasileira de
Assistencia aos Cancerosos (ABAC)
Hospital Mario Kroeff (H.M.K.)
Rua Magé no. 326 Penha Circular
20.000 Rio de Janeiro / Brazil

144

Mr. José Ermirio de Moraes Filho
(Chairman)
Fundaçao Antonio Prudente
P.O. Box 5271
Sao Paulo / Brazil

Dr. Antonio Franco Montoro
(President)
Grupo Brazileiro de Estudos
para Detecçao e Prevençao do Cancer
Hospital Oswaldo Cruz
Rua Joao Juliao 331
01323 Sao Paulo / Brazil

Prof. Carlos Aristides Maltez
(President)
Liga Bahiana contra o Cancer
Avenida D. Joao VI, no. 332
Brotas
40.000 Salvador-Bahia

Brazil

Dr. Edmur Flavio Pastorello (Dir.)
Divisao Nacional de Doenças
Cronico-Degenerativas -DNDCD-
Ministerio da Saude
Esplanada dos Ministerios
Bloco 11 -3o andar, sala 305
70.058 Brasilia, Distrito Federal
Brazil

Dr. Luiz Carlos Calmon Teixeira
(Secretary General)
Sociedade Brasileira de Cancerologia
Rua Humberto de Campos 11, Sala 803
40.000 Salvador-Bahia
Brazil

Bulgaria

Dr. G. Mitrov (President)
Bulgarian Oncological Society
U. Plovdivsko pole 6
Sofia-Darvenitza / Bulgaria

Canada

Dr. Robert A. Macbeth
(Executive Vice-President)
Canadian Cancer Society
130 Bloor Street West, Suite 1001
Toronto, Ontario M5S 2V7
Canada

Dr.David A. Boyes (Director)
Cancer Control Agency of
British Columbia
700-686 W. Broadway
Vancouver, British Columbia V5Z 1G1

Canada

Dr. Robert A. Macbeth
(Executive Director)
National Cancer Institute of Canada
130 Bloor Street West, Suite 1001
Toronto, Ontario M5S 2V7
Canada

Mr. Robert D. Gray
(Secretary.Treasurer)
The Ontario Cancer Treatment
and Research Foundation
7, Overlea Boulevard
Toronto, Ontario M4H 1A8

Canada

Chile

Dr. E. Raventos (Director)
Fundacion Arturo Lopez Pérez
Rancagua no. 878
Santiago / Chile

Liga Chilena contra el Cancer
Av. Pedro de Valdivia 3636
Casilla no. 15092 - Correo 11
Santiago / Chile

Ministerio de Salud Publica
Mac Iver 541
Santiago / Chile

China

Society of Oncology of
the Chinese Medical Association
c/o Dr. WU Huan hsing
Professor of Radiation Oncology
Director, Cancer Research Institute
Chinese Academy of Medical Sciences
Peking, / China

Colombia

Dr. Julio E. Ospina (Director)
Instituto Nacional de Cancerologia
Calle la, no. 9-85
Apartado Aereo 17158
Bogota / Colombia

Mrs. Maria Paulina Espinosa de Lopez
(President)
Liga Colombiana de Lucha contra el Cancer
Apartado Aéreo No. 057138   Cancer
Bogota / Colombia

Dr. German Jordan A. (President)
Sociedad Colombiana de Cancerologia
Carrera 13, no. 49-40
Edificio Marly -c.424
Casilla 105
Bogota, D.E. / Colombia

Cuba

Dr. Zoilo Marinello Vidaurreta (Dir.)
Instituto de Oncologia y Radiobiologia
del Ministerio de Salud Publica
Calle E y 29
Vedado
Habana / Cuba

Czechoslovakia

Czechoslovak Oncologic Society
Czechoslovak Medical Society J.E. Prukyne
Sokolska 31
Prague 2 / Czechoslovakia

Denmark

Mr. Ole Bang (Secretary Gen.)
Danish Cancer Society
Sólundsvej 1
2100 Copenhagen Ø / Denmark

Dominican Republic

Dr. Arturo Damiron R. (Director)
Instituto de Oncologia
"Doctor Heriberto Pieter"
Calle Bernardo Correa y Cidron no. 1
Santo Domingo, D.N.
Dominican Republic

Ecuador

Mr. Humberto Carbo Avellan
(President)
Sociedad de Lucha contra
el Cancer del Ecuador (SOLCA)
Casilla No. 3623
Guayaquil / Ecuador

Egypt

Prof. Salah Shahbander (Director)
Cancer Institute, Cairo University
Kasr El Aini Street
Fom El Kalig
Cairo / Egypt

Prof. Mahmoud M. Mahfous
(Chairman)
Kasr El-Einy Center of Radiation
Oncology and Nuclear Medicine
Kasr El-Einy, Cairo University Hospitals
Manial- Cairo / Egypt

Director General of
General Administration for Health
Foreign Relations
Ministry of Health
Cairo / Egypt

Mrs. Gehan Elsadat (President)
The Egyptian Cancer Society
174 Tahrir Street
Cairo / Egypt

Radiotherapy and Oncology Department
Faculty of Medicine
Alexandria University
Principal Hospital
Alexandria / Egypt

El Salvador

Dr. Narciso Diaz-Bazan
Instituto del Cancer
33 Avenida Norte y la Calle Pte.
San Salvador / El Salvador

Federal Republic of Germany

Prof. Fritz Linder (President)
Deutsche Krebsgesellschaft e.V.
c/o Chirurgische Universitätsklinik
Kirschnerstrasse 1
69 Heidelberg / Fed.Rep.of Germany

Prof. Dr. O. Westfhal (Director)
Deutsches Krebsforschungszentrum
Verwaltung
Im.Neuenheimer Feld 280
Postfach 101949
6900 Heidelberg 1

Fed.Rep. of Germany

Dr. G. Neumann (Secretary General)
Krebsverband Baden-Württemberg e.V.
Hohe Strasse 28
7000 Stuttgart 1 /Fed.Rep. of Germany

Westdeutsches Tumorzentrum.(WTZ)
Hufelandstrasse 55
4300 Essen 1/ fed. rep. of Germany

Finland

Mr. Niilo Voipio
(Secretary General)
Suomen Syöpäyhdistys
(The Cancer Society of Finland)
Liisankatu 21 B
00170 Helsinki 17/ Finland

France

Monsieur le Dr. J. Brugère
(Secretary General)
Association Française
pour l'Etude du Cancer
26 rue d'Ulm
75231 Paris Cédex 05 / France

Dr. Jacques Crozemarie (President)
Association pour le Développement de la
Recherche sur le Cancer à Villejuif
Boite Postale no. 3
94800 Villejuif / France

Prof. Claude Chardot (Director)
Centre Alexis Vautrin
Route Nationale 74, "Brabois"
54500 Vandoeuvre-les-Nancy / France

Prof. C.M. Lalanne (Director)
Centre Antoine Lacassagne
36,Voie Romaine
06054 Nice Cédex / France

Prof. P.F. Combes (Director)
Centre Claudius Regaud
11, rue Piquemil
31052 Toulouse Cédex / France

Prof. J.S. Abbatucci (Director)
Centre François Baclesse
Route de Lion sur Mer
14021 Caen Cédex / France

Prof. F. Cabanne (Director)
Centre Georges-François Leclerc
Centre Régional de Lutte contre
le Cancer de Bourgogne
Rue du Professeur Marion
21034 Dijon Cédex / France

Prof. Marcel Mayer (Director)
Centre Léon Bérard
28, rue Laënnec
69373 Lyon Cédex 2 / France

Prof. A. Demaille (Director)
Centre Oscar Lambret de Lille
Centre régional de Lutte contre
le Cancer de la Région Nord
Boite Postale no. 3569
59020 Lille Cédex / France

147

Dr. J. Gest (Director)
Centre René Huguenin de Lutte contre
le Cancer
5, rue Gaston Latouche
92211 Saint-Cloud / France

Prof. F. Larra (Director)
Centre régional Anticancéreux d'Angers
"Paul Papin"
2, rue Moll
49036 Angers Cédex / France

Prof. Y. Carcassonne (Director)
Centre régional de Lutte contre
le Cancer de Marseille
Institut J. Paoli - I. Calmettes
232, Boulevard de Sainte-Marguerite
13273 Marseille Cédex 2 / France

Prof. Claude Romieu (Director)
Centre régional de Lutte contre
le Cancer de Montpellier
Centre Paul Lamarque
2, avenue Bertin Sans
Boite Postale 5054
34033 Montpellier Cédex / France

Prof. Gaston Meyniel (Director)
Centre régional de Lutte contre le
Cancer Jean Perrin
Boite Postale 392
63011 Clermont-Ferrand Cédex

France

Dr. G. Methlin (Director)
Centre régional de Lutte contre le
Cancer "Paul Strauss"
3, rue de la Porte de l'Hôpital
67085 Strasbourg Cédex / France

Dr. R. Guihard (Director)
Centre régional de Lutte contre le
Cancer "René Gauducheau"
Quai Moncousu - Hotel-Dieu
44035 Nantes Cédex / France

Prof. J.L.Richier (Director)
Centre régional de Lutte Contre le Cancer
de Rennes
Centre anticancéreux - Pontchaillou
35011 Rennes / France

Mrs. B. Cheney (President)
Comité de la Savoie de la Ligue
nationale française contre le Cancer
3, Place Maché
73000 Chambéry / France

Mrs. Christiane Neys (President)
Comité de Paris
Ligue nationale française contre le Cancer
13, Avenue de la Grande Armée
75116 Paris / France

Dr. Gilbert Garnier (President)
Comité départemental de l'Aube
de la Ligue nationale contre le Cancer
43, rue Jaffiol
10150 Pont Sainte-Marie / France

Mrs. Ossude (President)
Comité départemental des Hauts-de-Seine
de la Ligue nationale française contre le Cancer
17, rue Raymond Barbet
92000 Nanterre / France

Mrs. Yvonne Baragué (President)
Comité départemental des Yvelines
de la Ligue nationale française contre le Cancer
41, rue de la Paroisse
78000 Versailles / France

Comité national français pour
les Relations avec l'UICC
c/o Fédération nationale des Centres de
Lutte contre le Cancer
101, rue de Tolbiac
75013 Paris / France

Prof. F. Cabanne (President)
Fédération nationale des Centres de
Lutte contre le Cancer
101, rue de Tolbiac
75013 Paris / France

Prof. Claude Lagarde (Dir.)
Fondation Bergonié
180, rue de Saint-Genès
33000 Bordeaux / France

Dr. R. Calle
Institut Curie
26, rue d'Ulm
75231 Paris Cédex 05 / France

Prof.G. Mathé (Director)
Institut de Cancérologie et
d'Immunogénétique (ICI)
et Service des Maladies Sanguines
Hôpital Paul-Brousse
14, Avenue Paul-Vaillant Couturier
94800 Villejuif / France

Prof. Pierre Denoix (Director)
Institut Gustave-Roussy
94805 Villejuif Cédex/ France

Prof. A. Cattan (Director)
Institut Jean-Godinot
1,Avenue du Général Koenig
B.P. 171
51056 Reims Cédex / France

Mr.R. Barmont
(Secretary General)
Ligue nationale française contre le Cancer
1-3 Avenue Stephen-Pichon
75013 Paris / France

Mr. Alexandre Oliva (President)*
Fédération nationale des Groupements
des Entreprises Françaises dans la Lutte
contre le Cancer
19A, rue Venture
13001 Marseille / France

German Democratic Republic

Prof. Dr.Stephan Tanneberger (Director)
Institut für Krebsforschung der
Akademie der Wissenschaften
der Deutschen Democratic Republic
Lindenberger Weg 80
1115 Berlin-Buch   German Democratic Rep

Greece

Mr.M. Konstantinidou (Secretary)
Aristotelian University
School of Medicine
Thessaloniki / Greece

Dr. B.Lisseos (President)
Hellenic Cancer Society
6, George Street
Kanigos Square
Athens 141 / Greece

Guatemala

Dr. Carlos Lizama Rubio (President)
Liga Nacional contra el Cancer de Guatemala
9a Calle No. 2-31, Zona 1
Guatemala / Guatemala

Honduras

Dr. Oscar Raudales Bara Hona
Liga Contra el Cancer
11 Ave S.O.
8a Calle .51
Barrio Supaya
San Pedro Sula / Honduras

Hong Kong

Dr. J.H.C. Ho (Chairman)
The Hong Kong Anti-Cancer Society
Nam Long Hospital
30, Nam Long Shan Road
Aberdeen / Hong Kong

Hungary

Egészségügyi Miniszterium
(Ministry of Health)
Akadémia u.10
Budapest V / Hungary

Iceland

Dr. G. Snaedal (President)
The Icelandic Cancer Society
P.O. Box 523
Reykjavik / Iceland

India

Dr. Jayasree Roy Chowdhury (Director)
Chittaranjan National Cancer Research
37, S.P. Mookerjee Road
Calcutta 700 026 / India

Dr. Usha B. Saraiya (Secretary)
Indian Academy of Cytologists
c/o Cytology Clinic
Cama & Albless Hospital
Mahapolika Marg
Bombay 400 001 / India

Dr. D.J. Jussawalla
(Honorary Secretary)
Indian Cancer Society
Dr. Ernest Borges Marg
Parel, Bombay 400 012 / India

Dr. M. Krishna Bhargava (Director)
Kidway Memorial Institute of Oncology
Hosur Road
Bangalore 560 029 / Karnataka

India

Dr.P.E. Desai (Director)
Tata Memorial Centre
Dr. Ernest Borges Marg
Parel, Bombay 400 012 / India

Dr. T.B. Patel (Director)
The Gujarat Cancer & Research Institute
New Civil Hospital Compound
Asarwa, Ahmedabad -380 016
Gujarat State / India

Dr. R.B. Patil (Director)
The Karnatak Cancer Therapy and
Research Institute
Hubli-Navanagar -580 025
Karnatak / India

Indonesia

Dr.W.M. Tamboenan (President)
Indonesian Cancer Society
Jl.Jendral S.Parman 82
Slipi
Jakarta / Indonesia

Dr.Sudarto Pringgoutomo
(Vice-Chairman)
Lembaga Kanker Indonesia
Jl. Dr.Sam Ratulangi 35
Djakarta Pusat/ Indonesia

Iran

Dr. T. Shariat-Madari(Director)
Cancer Institute
Iman Khomeiny Hospital
P.O. Box 14/1154
Teheran / Iran

Dr. A. Karamlou (Director)
Iran Cancer Organization
P.O. Box 13-511
Teheran 13 / Iran

Iraq

The Secretary General
Iraqi Cancer Society
P.O. Box 132
Baghdad / Iraq

Ireland

Lady Antonia Wardell
(Honorary Secretary)
Irish Cancer Society
5, Northumberland Road
Dublin 4 / Ireland

The Treasurer
Medical Research Council of Ireland
9, Clyde Road
Dublin 4 / Ireland

Israel

Mrs. Shoshana Eban (President)
Israel Cancer Association
P.O. Box 7065
Tel-Aviv / Israel

Italy

Prof. Giancarlo Maltoni
(Director)
Centro per lo Studio e la prevenzione
Oncologica /Unità Sanitaria Locale 10/E
Viale A. Volta 171
50131 Florence / Italy

Prof. Giovanni d'Errico
(Medical General Director)
Fondazione Senatore Pascale
Instituto Nazionale per la Prevenzione
lo Studio e la Cura dei Tumori
Via Mariano Semmola
80131 Naples / Italy

Dr. G. Palazzotto (Scientific Director)
Ente Ospedaliero Oncologico
"Maurizio Ascoli"
143 Via G. Parlavecchio
90127 Palermo / Italy

Prof. Vittorio Ventafridda
(Scientific Director)
Fondazione Floriani
Vicolo Fiori 2
20121 Milan / Italy

Dr. C. Biancifiori (Director)
Istituto di Anatomia e
Istologia Patologica
Divisione di Ricerche sul Cancro
Università degli Studi
06100 Perugia / Italy

Prof. Leonardo Santi (Director)
Istituto Scientifico per lo Studio
e la Cura dei Tumori
Viale Benedetto XV, 10-Pad. B.
16132 Genova / Italy

Dr.L. Caldarola (Director)
Istituto di Oncologia di Torino
Via Cavour 31
Turin 10123/ Italy

Prof. Umberto Veronesi (Director)
Istituto Nazionale per lo
Studio e la Cura dei Tumori
Via Venezian 1
20133 Milan / Italy

Dr. Michele Riolo (President)
Istituto Regina Elena per lo
Studio e la Cura dei Tumori
Viale Regina Elena 295
00161 Rome / Italy

Dr. Domenico Stalteri (Secr. Gen.)
Lega Italiana per la Lotta
contro i Tumori
Via Alessandro Torlonia 15
00161 Rome / Italy

Societa Italiana di Cancerologia
Via Venezian 1
20133 Milan / Italy

Dr. Guido Venosta (President)
Associazione Italiana per la
Ricerca sul Cancro *
Via Durini 5
20122 Milan / Italy

Dr.Katsuo Takeda (President)
Hokkaido Cancer Society
Kita 3 Nishi 12
Sapporo 060 / Japan

Prof. S. Garattini (Director)
Istituto di Ricerche Farmacologiche
"Mario Negri" *
Via Eritrea 62
20157 Milan / Italy

The Director
Institute for Cancer Research
Okayama University Medical School
Shikada-cho
Okayama 700 / Japan

Dr. E. Anglesio (Director)
Registro dei Tumori per il Piemonte e la
Valle d'Aosta *
Via Lagrange 2
10123 Turin / Italy

Mr. Koichi Nagashima
(General Secretary)
Japan Cancer Society
7th floor, Asahi Building
Ginza 6-6-7, Chuo-ku
Tokyo / Japan

Jamaica

Mr. D. Miller
(Permanent Secretary)
Ministry of Health and Environmental
P.O.Box 478   Control
Kingston / Jamaica

Office of the Director
Japanese Foundation for Cancer Research
c/o Cancer Institute
Kami-Ikebukuro 1-37-1
Toshima-ku, Tokyo 170 / Japan

Japan

Dr. Takeo Nagayo
Director of Research Institute
Aichi Cancer Center
81, Kanokoden Tashiro-cho
Chikusa-ku
Nagoya 464 / Japan

Mr.Mitsutaro Watanabe
Japanese Foundation for
Multidisciplinary Treatment of Cancer
3-2 Yotsuya, Shinjuku-ku
Tokyo 160 / Japan

Mr. Seigo Fukuma (Director)
Chiba Cancer Center
666-2 Nitona
Chiba
Chiba / Japan 280

Dr. Shoichi Yamagata (President)
Miyagi Cancer Society
Kamisugi 6 chome
Sendai 980 / Japan

Mr. Tatsuaki Hisano
Fukuoka Cancer Society
Chiyoda Seimei Nakasu Bldg.
4-17 Nakasu 5-chome
Hakata-ku, Fukuoka 810 /Japan

Dr. Shichiro Ishikawa (President)
National Cancer Center
Tsukiji 5-chome
Chuo-ku, Tokyo 104 / Japan

Mr. Shigeru Sawada
(Executive Director)
Osaka Taigan Kyokai
Osaka Association Against Cancer
c/o Osaka Asahi Shimbun Sha
Nakanoshima 3-2-4
Kita-ku,Osaka 530 / Japan

Mrs. Fujiko Iwasaki (President)
Princess Takamatsu Cancer Research Fund
Room 505, 1-25 Nishi Azabu 3-chome
Minatoku, Tokyo 106 /Japan

Dr. Seiichi Yoshida (President)
Saitama Cancer Center
Ina-machi, Kitaadachi-gun
Saitama-ken 362 / Japan

Mr. Kunio Yoshioka
(Secretary General)
Science Council of Japan
22-34 Roppongi, 7-chome
Minato-ku, Tokyo 106 / Japan

Dr. Nobuyuki Senda (President)
The Center for Adult Diseases
Nakaimichi 1-chome
Higashinari-ku, Osaka 537 / Japan

Mr. Keiji Iwata
(Vice-Chairman, Board of Directors)
The Children's Cancer Association of Japan
2-4-11 Nishi-Shimbashi
Minato-ku, Tokyo 105 / Japan

Dr. Haruo Sugano
(Secretary General)
The Japanese Association for Cancer Research
c/o Cancer Institute
Kami-Ikebukuro 1-37-1
Toshima-ku, Tokyo 170 / Japan

Mr.Kazumasa Masubuchi,M.D.
President
The Japan Society for
Cancer Therapy
Second Surgical Division
Kyoto University Medical School
54,Shogoin-kawaracho
Sakyo-ku
Kyoto 606   Japan

Dr. Reiji Natori (President)
The Jikei University School of Medicine
3-25-8 Nishi-Shimbashi
Minato-ku, Tokyo 105 / Japan

Jordan

Dr. Ibrahim Shami (President)
The Jordanian Cancer Society
P.O. Box 86 Tal 65131
Amman

Jordan

Ministry of Health
P.O. Box 86
Amman / Jordan

Kenya

Dr.J.N. Onyango
Cancer Council of Kenya *
c/o Radiotherapy Department
Kenyatta National Hospital
Box 20723
Nairobi / Kenya

Korea

Dr. Suk Whan Kim (President)
Korean Cancer Society
c/o Chung Ang Hospital
Chung Ang Cancer Institute
161 Waryong-Dong
Chongno-Gu
Seoul 110 / Korea

Kuwait

Dr. Nail El Naquib
(Under-Secretary)
Ministry of Public Health
P.O. Box 5
Kuwait / Kuwait

Lebanon

Dr. Philip A. Salem
Lebanese Cancer Society
c/o American University Hospital
P.O. Box 113-6044
Beirut / Lebanon

Liberia

Dr. A.O. Sobo
(2nd Vice-President)
Liberian Cancer Society
P.O. Box 3605
Monrovia / Liberia

Luxembourg
Dr. E. Duhr
Ministère de la Santé publique
et de l'Environnement
57, Boulevard de la Pétrusse
Luxembourg / Luxembourg

Malaysia

Dr. S.K. Dharmalingham
(Vice-President)
The National Cancer Society of Malaysia
P.O.Box 2187
Kuala Lumpur / Malaysia

Malta

Dr. Alf Grech
(Chief Government Medical Officer)
Department of Health *
15 Merchants Street
Valletta / Malta

Mexico

Secretaria de Salubridad y Asistencia
Officina de Asuntos Internacionales
Reforma y Lieja
México, D.F. / Mexico

Dr. José Noriega Limon (Director)
Instituto Nacional de Cancerologia *
San Fernando 22
Tlalpan
Mexico 22, D.F. / Mexico

Dr. German Garcia (Director)
Servicio de Enfermedades Neoplasicas *
Spanish Hospital
Av. Ejercito Nacional 613
Mexico, D.F./ Mexico

Morocco

Prof. Y. Boutaleb
(Secretary General)
Association Marocaine pour la Lutte
contre le Cancer, A.M.L.C.
B.P. 589
Casablanca / Morocco

Namibia (South West Africa)

Mr. T.F.J. van Aardt (Secretary)
The Cancer Association of
South West Africa-Namibia
P.O. Box 30230
Pionierspark 9112
Windhoek / Namibia

The Netherlands

Dr. Zwanette M. Beekman
(Director)
Koningin Wilhelmina Fonds - Nederlands
Organisatie voor de Kankerbestrijding
Sophialaan 8-10
1075 BR Amsterdam /The Netherlands

Ministry of Public Health
and Environmental Hygiene
Dokter Reijersstraat 12
Leidschendam /The Netherlands

Prof. Dr.F.J. Cleton
(Scientific Director)
The Netherlands Cancer Institute
Plesmanlaan 121
1066 CX Amsterdam /The Netherlands

New Zealand

Dr.J. Murphy (Secretary)
Cancer Society of New Zealand
P.O. Box 10340
Wellington, C.1
New Zealand

Nigeria

Dr. G.C. Ejeckam (Vice-President)
Cancer Society of Nigeria
P.O. Box 2205
Enugu / Nigeria

Dr. D.O.S. Ajayi (Hon.Secretary)
Nigerian Cancer Society
c/o Department of Radiation Biology
and Radiotherapy
Lagos Univ. Teaching Hospital
P.M.B 12003 Lagos / Nigeria

Norway

Mr. Ottar S. Jacobsen
(Secretary General)
Norwegian Cancer Society
Huitfeldtsgt 49
Oslo 2 / Norway

Mrs. Lilly Christensen
(Secretary-General)
Norwegian Society for Fighting Cancer
Kongenst. 6
Oslo 1 / Norway

Pakistan

Dr. Munir Ahmed Siddiqui (Dir.)
Atomic Energy Medical Centre
Liaquat Medical College & Hospital
Jamshoro / Pakistan

Dr. Gul Rahman (Dir.)
Institute of Radiotherapy and
Nuclear Medicine (IRNUM)
University Campus
Feshawar / Pakistan

Ministry of Health
Social Welfare and Population
Health and Social Welfare Division
Government of Pakistan
Islamabad / Pakistan

Dr. Mahfooz Akhtar
Nuclear Medicine Centre
P.O. Box No. 5
Larkana / Pakistan

Panama

Mrs. Isabel J. de Nunez
(President)
Asociacion Nacional contra el Cancer
Apartado Postal 7358
Panama 5 / Panama

Paraguay

Prof. M. Riveros
Instituto Nacional del Cancer
Sebastian Gaboto 495
Asuncion / Paraguay

Peru

Miss. F. Heller (President)
Fundacion Peruana de Cancer
Casilla 4408
Lima / Peru

Dr. Eduardo Caceres (Director)
Instituto Nacional de Enfermedades Neoplasicas
Avenida Alfonso Ugarte 825
Lima / Peru

Sr.Antero Aspillaga (President)
Liga Peruana de Lucha contra el Cancer
Jr. Chancay 922 Of. 1
Lima / Peru

Philippines

Dr. Tranquilino Elicano (President)
National Cancer Control Center (NCCC)
San Lazaro Compound
Rizal Avenue
Sta. Cruz
Manila / Philippines

Dr. Constantino P. Manahan (President)
Philippine Cancer Society, Inc.
310 San Rafael St., San Miguel
Manila 2804 / Philippines

Poland

Prof. Dr. Leszek Wozniak (President)
The Polish Oncological Society
Ul. Gagarina 4
93-509 Lodz /Poland

Portugal

Prof. José Conde (Director)
Instituto Portugues de Oncologia
de Francisco Gentil
Rua Prof. Lima Basto
Lisbon 4 /Portugal

Dr. Gentil Martins (Secretary General)
Liga Portuguesa Contra o Cancro
Rua Prof. Edmundo Lima Basto
Palhava
1093 Lisboa Codex /Portugal

Romania

Dr.O. Costachel (President)
Société d'Oncologie de Roumanie
Str.Dr. Félix 54
P.B. 5916
62 Bucharest /Roumanie

Singapore

The Chairman
The Singapore Cancer Society
16/K L Realty Center
Enggor Street
Singapore 0207 / Singapore

South Africa

Mr.J.P.F.Delport
(National Secretary)
The National Cancer Association
of South Africa
P.O. Box 2000
Johannesburg 2000/ South Africa

Spain

Dr. J.J. Tafalla Sampietro
(Executive Director)
Asociacion Espanola contra el Cancer
Amador de los Rios 5
Madrid 4 / Spain

Sri-Lanka

Prof. H.V.J. Fernando (President)
Sri-Lanka Cancer Society *
37/25 Bullers Lane
Colombo 7 / Sri-Lanka

Sweden

Mrs. Ejda Wesslén
The Cancer Society of Stockholm
Radiumhemmet
104 01 Stockholm /Sweden

Mrs. Dagmar von Walden-Laing
(Executive Director)
The Swedish Cancer Society
Sturegatan 14
114 36 Stockholm / Sweden

Switzerland

Schweizerische Krebsliga
Monbijoustrasse 61
Postfach 2284
3001 Bern / Switzerland

Syria

The Secretariat
Syrian Cancer Society
B.P. 4567
Damascus / Syria

Thailand

The President
Thai Cancer Society
1909/86 Soi Ruam Patana
Charunsanitwong Road
Bangplud, Bangkoknoi
Dhonburi / Thailand

Trinidad

Dr. A. Cuthbert
The Trinidad and Tobago Cancer Society
157a Western Main Road
St. James / Trinidad and Tobago

Tunisia

Prof. N. Mourali
Institut Salah Azaiz
Bab Saadoun
Tunis / Tunisia

Turkey

Dr. Erdogan Inal
Aid Organisation of Ankara
Oncology Hospital
Baskanligi
Etimesgut
Ankara / Turkey

Dr. Zülfü Sami Ozgen (President)
National Federation Against Cancer
Lobut Sok. no.61
Sishane-Istanbul / Turkey

Dr. D. Firat (President)
Türk Kanser Arastirma ve Savas Kurumu
(The Turkish Association for Cancer
Research and Control)
P.K. 1078
Yenisehir, Ankara / Turkey

Union of Soviet Socialist Republics

Ministerstvo Zdravochranenia SSSR
Rachmanovsky pereulok 3
Moscow / USSR

United Kingdom

Dr. M.J. Embleton
(Honorary Secretary)
British Association for Cancer Research
c/o Cancer Research Campaign Laboratories
University Park
Nottingham NG7 2RD / U. K.

Brigadier K.D. Gribbin
(Secretary General)
Cancer Research Campaign
2 Carlton House Terrace
London SW1Y 5AR / U.K.

Prof. L.G. Lajtha
Christie Hospital and Holt
Radium Institute
Manchester M20 9BX / U.K.

Mr. A.B.L. Clarke (Secretary)
Imperial Cancer Research Fund
P.O. Box no. 123
Lincoln's Inn Fields
London WC2A 3PX / U.K.

Dr. Robin Weiss (Director)
Institute of Cancer Research:
Royal Cancer Hospital
34 Sumner Place, Fulham Road
London SW7 3NU / U.K.

Mr. R.L. Davison
Executive Director
Manchester Regional Committee
for Cancer Education
Kinnaird Road
Manchester,M 20 9QL

U.K.

Mr. Paul A. Sturgess
(Secretary)
Marie Curie Memorial Foundation
124 Sloane Street
London SW1X 9BP

U.K.

Mr. Michael Downs
(Org. Secretary)
Tenovus
111 Cathedral Road
Cardiff CF1 9PH / U.K.

Mr. M.A. Wood (Director)
Ulster Cancer Foundation
40 Eglantine Avenue
Belfast BT9 60X / U.K.

Prof. Norman Cromwell
Eppley Cancer Institute
42nd and Dewey Avenue
Omaha, Nebraska 68105/ U.S.A.

United States of America

Dr. Frederick S. Philips
(Secretary Treasurer)
American Association
for Cancer Research Inc.
1275 York Avenue
New York, N.Y. 10021 / U.S.A.

Dr. Joseph G. Fortner (President)
General Motors Cancer
Research Foundation, Inc.
767 Fifth Avenue
New York, N.Y. 10022 /U.S.A.

Mr. Lane W. Adams
(Executive Vice-President)
American Cancer Society, Inc.
777 Third Avenue
New York, N.Y. 10017 /U.S.A.

Dr. Ch.A. LeMaistre (President)
M.D. Anderson Hospital and Tumor Institute
The University of Texas
Texas Medical Center
Houston, Texas 77030 /U.S.A.

Dr. E.A. Mirand
(Secretary Treasurer)
Association of American
Cancer Institutes
c/o Roswell Park Memorial Institute
666 Elm Street
Buffalo, N.Y. 14263 /U.S.A.

Dr. Lewis Thomas (President)
Memorial Sloan-Kettering Cancer Center
1275 York Avenue
New York, N.Y.10021/ U.S.A.

Dr. Anthony P. Monaco
(Scientific Director)
Cancer Research Institute
New England Deaconess Hospital
185 Pilgrim Road
Boston, Mass. 02215 / U.S.A.

The Michigan Cancer Foundation
110 East Warren Avenue
Detroit, Michigan 48201/ U.S.A.

Mr. David W. Walsh
(Secretary and Executive Director)
Damon Runyon-Walter Winchell Cancer
33 West 56th Street   Fund
New York, N.Y. 10019/ U.S.A.

Dr. Stanley G. Parry
Northern California Cancer Programme
1801 Page Mil Road, Bldg.B, s.200
Palo Alto
California 94304 / U.S.A.

Dr. Oscar N. Guerra
Ellis Fischel State Cancer
Hospital and Cancer Research Center
Business Loop 70 & Garth Avenue
Columbia, Missouri 65201 /U.S.A.

Dr. G.P. Murphy (Director)
Roswell park Memorial Institute
666 Elm Street
Buffalo, N.Y.14263/ U.S.A.

Dr. Alvin M. Mauer (Director)
St. Jude Children's Research Hospital
332 North Lauderdale, P.O.Box 318
Memphis, TN 38101/ U.S.A.

Dr. A.G. Knudson, Jr. (President)
The Fox Chase Cancer Center
7701 Burholme Avenue
Fox Chase
Philadelphia, Pa. 19111/ U.S.A.

Dr. William Hutchinson
(President and Director)
The Fred Hutchinson Cancer
Research Center
1124 Columbia Street
Seattle, Wa. 98104/ U.S.A.

Mrs. June Ewing (Executive Secretary)
U.S.A. National Committee on UICC
National Research Council
2101 Constitution Avenue
Washington, D.C. 20418/ U.S.A

Uruguay

Prof. H. Kasdorf
Departamento de Oncologia
Hospital de Clinicas
"Dr. Manuel Quintela"
Avenida Italia, Casilla de Correo 930
Montevideo / Uruguay

Venezuela

Dr. Aquiles Erminy R. (Director)
Direccion de Oncologia /Ministerio de
Sanidad y Asistencia Social
Avenida los Proceres Cruce
con Calle Oriente
Quinta A.Tito No. 1
San Bernardino / Venezuela

Dr. Ruben Merenfeld (President)
Sociedad Anticancerosa de Venezuela
Apartado de Correos 6702
Canonigos a Esperanza 43
Caracas 101 / Venezuela

Dr. J.A. Ravelo Celis (President)
Sociedad Venezolana de Oncologia
Apartado Postal 70.398
Caracas 107 / Venezuela

Yugoslavia

Mr. Rade Kusic (President)
Drustvo Srbije Za Borbu Protiv Raka
(The Society for the Fight
Against Cancer of Serbia)
Knez Mihajlova 2/VI
Belgrade / Yugoslavia

Prof. I. Padovan (President)
Liga Za Borbu Protiv Raka SR Hrvatske
(The Society for the Fight
Against Cancer of Croatia)
Ilica 197
41000 Zagreb / Yugoslavia

Dr. Nenad Markovic (President)
Zdruzenie na Lekarite od Makedonija
(Yugoslav Society of Cancerology)
ul. Dame Gruev br. 3
91000 Skopje / Yugoslavia

Zimbabwe

Mr. Nehemiah Munyoro (Secretary)
The Cancer Association Zimbabwe *
Mpilo Central Hospital
P.O. Box 2096
Bulawayo / Zimbabwe

OTHER UICC PUBLICATIONS RELATED TO
HEALTH EDUCATION ABOUT CANCER

Influencing Smoking Behaviour. Technical Report Series Vol. 3.
Edited by J. Wakefield, 1969. 90 pp. Free. ISBN 92-9018-003-X.

Teoría y práctica de la educación sanitaria en la lucha contra el
cáncer - Recopilación de trabajos originales. Serie de Informes
Técnicos de la UICC Volumen 10. Obra publicada por el Comité de
Educación del Público de la Unión Internacional contra el Cáncer.
1974. 123 pp. Free.

Public Education About Cancer - Recent Research and Current
Programmes. Technical Report Series Vol. 26. Edited by
J. Wakefield, 1977. 103 pp. Free.ISBN 92-9018-026-9.

International Catalogue of Films, Filmstrips and Slides on
Public Education about Cancer. Trilingual edition (English,
French, Spanish). Technical Report Series Vol. 29. 1977.
518 pp. Swiss Francs 60.- ISBN 92-9018-029-3.

Public Education About Cancer - Recent Research and Current
Programmes. Technical Report Series Vol. 31. Edited by
J. Wakefield, 1978. 96 pp. Swiss Francs 20.- ISBN 92-9018-031-5.

Cancer Education in Schools - A Guidebook for Teachers. Technical
Report Series Vol. 38. 1978. 116 pp. Swiss Francs 32.-
ISBN 92-9018-038-2. First Reprinting 1981.
Information about the translation of this Manual in Arabic,
Chinese, Danish, Finnish, French, German, Italian, Norwegian,
Polish, Portuguese, Serbo-Croat and Spanish is available from
the UICC Geneva Office.

Involving Doctors in Health Education about Cancer. Technical
Report Series Vol. 44. Edited by D.J. Hill, M.W. Heffernan
and D.I. Rice, 1979. 116 pp. Swiss Francs 20.- ISBN 92-9018-044-7.

Public Education About Cancer - Recent Research and Current
Programmes. Technical Report Series Vol. 45. Edited by P. Hobbs,
1979. 104 pp. Swiss Francs 20.- ISBN 92-9018-045-5.

Slide Compilation of Cancer Control Posters. Technical Report
Series Vol. 46. Prepared under the auspices of the UICC Programme
on Cancer Campaign and Organization, 1979. 51 pp. Swiss Francs
32.- ISBN 92-9018-046-3.

Guidelines for Smoking Control. Technical Report Series Vol. 52
(revised edition of the UICC Technical Report Series Vol. 28).
Edited by N. Gray and M. Daube, 1980. 172 pp. Swiss Francs 24.-
ISBN 92-9018-052-8.
Information about the translation of this Manual in Spanish
is available from the UICC Geneva Office.

International Catalogue of Films, Filmstrips and Slides on
Public Education about Cancer (First Supplement). Trilingual
edition (English, French, Spanish). Technical Report Series
Vol. 54. 1980. 187 pp. Swiss Francs 44.- ISBN 92-9018-054-4.

Public Education About Cancer - Recent Research and Current Programmes. Technical Report Series Vol. 55. Edited by P. Hobbs, 1980. 101 pp. Swiss Francs 20.- ISBN 92-9018-055-2.

Public Education About Cancer - Recent Research and Current Programmes. Technical Report Series Vol. 62. Edited by P. Hobbs, 1981. 87 pp. Swiss Francs 20.- ISBN 92-9018-062-5.

Slide Compilation of Cancer Control Posters. (First Supplement). Technical Report Series Vol. 64. Prepared under the auspices of the UICC Programme on Cancer Campaign and Organization, 1982. 67 pp. (Illus.). Swiss Francs 36.- ISBN 92-9018-064-1.

Public Education About Cancer - Recent Research and Current Programmes. Technical Report Series Vol. 67. Edited by P. Hobbs, 1982. 104 pp. Swiss Francs 20.- ISBN 92-9018-067-6.

Orders should be placed with : Hans Huber Publishers
                                76 Länggassstrasse
                                3000 Bern 9
                                Switzerland

Notes

Notes

Notes

Printed in Switzerland
by
Imprimerie W. Gassmann SA, Bienne